# THE ART OF
# DOCTORING

## MOYEZ JIWA

Published in Australia by Perceptive Press
theartofdoctoring.com

National Library of Australia Publication Data
available via www.nla.gov.au

ISBN: 978-0-9944328-3-4

Printed in Australia

Cover & Book Design: Reese Spykerman
Interior Layout: Kelly Exeter

10 9 8 7 6 5 4 3 2 1

First Edition

*For Bernadette, who has been helping me to give back for thirty years and counting.*

*And for Adam, Kieran and Matthew—*
*you can make a difference.*

# CONTENTS

# INTRODUCTION

We eat too much, drink too much alcohol and are far too sedentary. For many of us, a lifetime of such habits leads to long-term poor health—often sooner rather than later.

What's more, we have less effective healthcare and pay more for it than necessary.

So far, our efforts to improve the outcomes of visiting a doctor have been disappointing, perhaps because we haven't been focusing on the fundamental reason people seek help from a doctor.

When we're sick, we want relief from our discomfort, whether it's physical or psychological. But while a one-size-fits-all medication or procedure may be convenient it often fails, is becoming increasingly unaffordable and in some cases can actually be harmful. And the outcomes in countries that spend substantially more per capita on healthcare (most notably the United States) are no better than in countries that spend proportionally less.

This book focuses on how we can improve those outcomes globally by answering a number of questions:

- How can we help sick people get better and increase their participation and satisfaction in their own healthcare, without yet another round of ineffective government policy 'reforms'?
- How do we make the most of our limited resources (especially in family medicine) when a generation or more of researchers and policymakers has failed?
- How can we harness what's already available to help doctors empower their patients to get well?
- How do we encourage doctors to be more creative and serve people more effectively?
- How can we relieve the pressure on the system by engaging the most underutilised and creative resources—the doctors, their staff and the people who need their help—in healthcare design?

In outlining my perspective, I make one major assertion: that every doctor can make a huge difference to the outcomes for their patients simply by paying close attention to how they practice the art of doctoring.

My goal in writing this book is to offer hope and to inspire individual doctors (especially medical students) to become healers rather than technicians.

> "Finding a good doctor is like finding a good lover:
> there are lots of anecdotes but no data."
> —Richard Smith[1]

The first of August is the worst day to end up in hospital in Ireland. That's the first day for all newly qualified doctors, which is a mixture of hope and fear.

I can still remember my first day. I donned my newly laundered white coat, pocketed my stethoscope and drug formulary and grabbed the Parker pen gifted to me by my proud parents. Fully equipped and more than a little terrified, I headed through the swing doors into the surgical ward where I'd spend the first three months of my internship. Little did I know, as I stood on the threshold of the huge public hospital as a newly minted doctor, that I already had everything I needed to get me through my career as a doctor.

I was met by Eileen Dorley, the nurse in charge. 'Good morning Doctor,' she said enthusiastically.

It was the first time anyone had called me 'Doctor.' It's a hard-won moment no doctor ever forgets.

'Good morning Sister,' I replied, as that's what the nurse in charge was called back then. 'What can I do first this morning?'

'Well Doctor,' she said. 'You could start by prescribing antiemetics for the patients going to the operating theatre later today.'

I reached for the drug formulary in my hip pocket and hesitated for a moment—my training had taught me there were lots of possibilities—then asked the still smiling Sister Dorley the name of the professor's preferred antiemetic.

'That would be Stemetil, Doctor!' she beamed.

I clicked my pen and pulled up the first prescription. I started to spell the word aloud as I wrote: 'S-T-E...'

'M-E-T-I-L,' she completed.

'Thank you, Sister. And what dose does he like to use?'

'Twelve point five milligrams twice a day Doctor,' she replied. 'Just tick the "6am" and "6pm" boxes. The rest Doctor,' she said while inclining her head slightly, 'is written on your name badge.' She said it without a hint of sarcasm or unkindness.

In the three months that followed, Eileen Dorley made it her mission to help me transition from graduate to doctor.

Despite many gruelling days on call, with the help of her nursing team I found time to publish my research in an international journal. That publication, and the reference from the professor, helped me secure my spot on one of the most prestigious specialist training schemes in the UK.

I owe a great deal to Eileen Dorley. She demonstrated the value of seeing patients and young doctors within the context of their lives, anticipating their needs and responding with kindness. She also taught me that supposedly less qualified people could help me become a better doctor as long as I was open to practicing with humility.

I've often wondered what people want in a doctor and whether doctors are trained to deliver it. Michael Boland summarised the typical research findings about patient sentiment in 1995[2]: 'Surprisingly few people seem to worry about the technical competence of doctors. What they worry about is their doctor's ability to understand the patient as a person and provide the right guidance.' Former *British Medical Journal* editor Richard Smith, whom I quoted earlier, was probably right in saying there is no data about what makes a good doctor.

A doctor is someone whose patients are likely to share their secrets, worries and hopes with. Someone they trust with their lives. In light of this, we might evaluate a doctor much like Alison Siegel advised women to evaluate a first date[3].

Was he nice to the servers?

Did he talk about himself the whole time?

Did you laugh?

Did he check his phone?

Did you feel chemistry?

Was he a good listener?

Based on Siegel's list, it seems people will invest in relationships when they believe the other person is:

- respectful
- willing and able to give their undivided attention
- humble
- genuinely interested

In medicine a doctor, as one of the parties on 'the date' may have the required qualifications. But they still need to be curious about the context of any symptoms. To be invited to continue the relationship they must be a focused and attentive listener.

In a medical consultation interest in the patient isn't limited to their medical history, allergies or genetic profile. It can also include their personal circumstances. Perhaps the patient has recently moved to the area, changed jobs, rented a new home, or experienced other stressful life events (e.g. death, divorce, job loss).

Good doctors treat the whole patient and anticipate that the person's current discomfort may be rooted in this context. Doctors look beyond the presenting illness and factor in the support required alongside any prescribed treatment.

If you feel as I do, then you probably believe the best doctors cultivate trusting relationships that lead to better treatment and patient outcomes. When we consult a doctor, we value eye contact. We want them to listen closely, pick up on verbal and non-verbal cues and be respectful. But above all, we want them to be uncompromising in their conviction that our perspective as the person who believes they are sick is the one that matters most.

Good doctors constantly remind themselves that people are free to make choices. The best doctors see their role as advisers and advocates rather than all-knowing experts. We want to know they will always have our best interests at heart.

Anatole Broyard expresses it like this:

> *What do I want in a doctor? I would say that I want one who is a close reader of illness and a good critic of medicine.... I see no reason or need for my doctor to love me, nor would I expect him to suffer with me. I wouldn't demand a lot of my doctor's time, I just wish he would brood on my situation for perhaps five minutes, that he would give me his whole mind only once, be bonded with me for a brief space, survey my soul as well as my flesh, to get at my illness, for each man is ill in his own way.[4]*

Many people who visit a doctor may have symptoms or need help with something, but they are not actually sick let alone dying. And yet they may be prescribed drugs they don't need, offered tests that aren't warranted and referred to specialists for no benefit. (I'll be exploring the reasons for this later in this book.)

While people can be nudged to make different choices, doctors assume their patients can make difficult decisions based only on information they receive from someone armed with a stethoscope. Many doctors' attempts at persuading us to eat less, exercise more, drink less alcohol and stop smoking are weak because they talk only about the harmful effects of our poor choices.

Those who fund healthcare, be they insurers or government, their favourite ploy is to give health practitioners an incentive to 'educate' us using this impersonal data. To help solve this healthcare crisis I suggest deploying the creativity and connection of healthcare practitioners with patients. If we don't, practitioners will become (and perhaps remain) part of the problem.

We know family doctors deliver 90% of healthcare, with the bulk of their work centred around advice rather than intervention. We also know doctors are more dissatisfied with their working conditions than ever before, and some are reporting record rates of burnout. People often ignore the fact that doctors can't perform miracles to reverse the consequences of their poor choices. At the same time, patients are treated as if their expectations and demands are partly to blame for the healthcare sector struggling.

Unfortunately, government investment in primary care (the first port of call for patients who think they're sick) doesn't influence voters. They're more impressed with the unveiling of a new hospital stocked with state-of-the-art equipment and facilities. They don't appreciate how empowering them to make better lifestyle choices leads to better health outcomes. Instead they choose (or are forced) to deal with the consequences of their choices when they arise.

Patients are becoming increasingly disillusioned with medicine. For most people, access to decent healthcare is a significant concern. But they're largely served by a healthcare sector driven by efficiency and profit.

Healthcare has become a business where 'wellbeing' is a commodity, framed by how much we access and then consume the products of commercial biomedicine. People are told their health problems can be solved with supplements, drugs or procedures. Our personal healthcare data is used to paint a more compelling picture of our apparent morbidity. As a consequence, while the healthcare industry solves problems for some people, it can cause problems for those who opt for treatments they don't need or that prove to be harmful. In OECD countries, hospitals spend one in every six dollars treating the side-effects of medicines.[5]

I believe these problems are partly due to fact that the art of doctoring—the connection between the doctors and their patients—isn't being used to full effect. It's far more convenient to offer someone a pill than to deal with the poor behaviour at the heart of their problem.

Governments worldwide have spent billions on large-scale reform to try and improve measurable outcomes. History is littered with disappointing and abandoned attempts to get more for every healthcare dollar. In the UK the 'big idea' was fundholding, then primary care trusts and then the Quality Outcomes Framework. In the US it was the Affordable Care Act. And in Australia it was divisions of general practice, then Medicare locals and now Primary Health Care Networks. But none of these ideas seem to have improved outcomes or saved money, so think tanks have recommended further radical policy change.

Hardly any of these reforms effectively mobilised the creativity or insight of healthcare professionals. None of them appear to consider the perspective of the consumer who may have better options, depending on how they explain their problem to their doctor. Someone with a viral upper respiratory tract infection wants to feel better, not to have the microbe chemically wiped from their body (especially given that right now it's technically impossible). Healthcare professionals are often cast as technicians and bureaucrats working with a paying customer rather than people who can reframe problems and generate more effective solutions.

In every other commercial setting, the focus tends to be on improving the customer experience. In a world of infinite choices, the success of any business or brand relies on delivering an experience that delights its customers. The best brands are built around a synergy between employees and customers that reflects the company's mission.

A synergy that's missing in most subsidised healthcare settings. What can be done to solve this problem? The answer is hidden in plain sight. We need to revisit what happens during the consultation and make the most of those precious minutes when doctors engage patients face to face.

Despite the gloomy predictions about healthcare's higher costs and lower quality, doctors can and should be involved in reforming our ailing health systems. Rather than relying on policymakers to provide additional revenues and policies to optimise outcomes, doctors can and should create the change we all want to see for ourselves. We've known how to fix many of our healthcare challenges for decades. By using the resourceful communities of healthcare practitioners, we can solve many of them ourselves. What difference could this attention to detail make to patients?

In an overburdened and increasingly bureaucratised system, these details are considered optional rather than essential. Doctors tend to focus entirely on the technical aspects of the consultation—ordering tests and prescribing from a formulary—as if the reason people seek help hardly matters at all.

Of course, nothing could be further from the truth. If the past few decades have taught us anything about human behaviour it's that people can be trusted to make the best choice when they're ill, providing they are appropriately guided and take their circumstances into account.

Much of what I offer in this book is based on how we perform rituals in healthcare. In medicine we need to develop consultation rituals similar to those surgeons perform before they deploy their scalpel on the patient's skin. We need to consider every interaction between the two key performers on that private stage known as the doctor's office—the greeting, the seating and the meeting—and develop rituals to improve the outcome for everyone involved, including those who pay for the encounter. I frame this 'art of doctoring' within what I've dubbed 'the Theatre Model©', where every element of the encounter between patient and doctor is defined, and their role in the success of that encounter is carefully considered.

Let's begin.

# 1

# FOURTEEN STORIES THAT TAUGHT ME
## *The Art of Doctoring*

Doctors learn and relate their experiences through stories. In this chapter I'll be telling 14 stories about people who inspired this book.

In a typical day a family doctor will consult a similar number of people with broadly similar problems. Some of these stories relate to my patients, while others have been shared by friends or family. (In each case their details have been changed to protect their privacy.)

I'll be referring to these people by their pseudonyms throughout the book and recalling their cases by the 'problem' in brackets after their name. I'm not suggesting people should be reduced to one issue. It will simply make it easier for me to refer to them in later chapters.

# Pauline and Mick (pneumonia)

## *The backstory*

Pauline and Mick were in their late 70s and had a myriad of problems requiring regular visits to their family doctor. And for most of their married life they sought advice from Dr Irvine, who got to know them well over the years.

They were deeply fond of Dr Irvine. He was there when they faced the challenges of working on factory floors while trying to keep their young family fed. He was there for all four of Pauline's pregnancies. He'd turn up late at night in all weather (often stubbing out a cigarette as he pulled up) to examine a feverish child. And despite the limitations of medicine in the 60s and 70s, the family prospered in relatively good health.

But when Dr Irvine finally retired from his practice in the 1980s, everything changed for Pauline and Mick.

Home visits are a thing of the past, and not encouraged by the new managers of their healthcare provider. Pauline and Mick, who have never owned a car, now walk three kilometres to the clinic where they wait for up to an hour to see a doctor.

And the doctor they *do* see might know their diagnostic history, but not much else about them. (Or any of their patients, for that matter.) For instance, the doctor doesn't know Pauline's physical ailments often reflect her loss of self-worth after retiring from paid work a decade earlier.

## *The event*

One winter Pauline developed a fever and cough and made her way to the clinic. The deputy doctor examined her and without asking how she got to the clinic, told her to visit the hospital emergency department for a chest X-ray.

Pauline didn't feel up to using public transport, so she decided to go home that afternoon to rest. Next morning her grandson drove her and Mick to the hospital where they waited six hours to be seen by a physician.

### The outcome

Pauline was diagnosed with pneumonia and spent two weeks in hospital. When she finally got a bed in the hospital she was confused and breathless. Mick had no idea why his wife was so sick, or when she'd be well enough to come home. Two weeks later Pauline returned home in a taxi, still mildly confused and dizzy.

The medications she was taking were similar to those prescribed months before by her regular doctor. But despite them being discontinued due to side effects long before she was admitted, her prescription hadn't been updated in the practice records. The deputy who sent her to the emergency department listed the wrong drugs in his referral letter. And Pauline didn't notice because the letter had the chemical name rather than the brand name.

### The lesson

In many countries, family doctors don't know as much about their patients' life circumstances as they may have 30 or 40 years ago. Resources in the health service are also limited and it's unlikely more resources will be made available to service the needs of these patients. The proportion of people aged 65 or over is increasing, as is the proportion of people with long-term conditions.

Every interaction with Pauline and Mick needs to count. When Pauline presents with symptoms of a potentially life-limiting illness, she can't be put at further risk because of her clinician's blind spot to her circumstances. It's important to not only take appropriate action, but also to convey information in a way that ensures they know what action needs to be taken. On this occasion, the failures were mainly to do with communication.

Pauline made a full recovery and went back to planning her next trip to see her grandchildren overseas. But unsatisfactory healthcare experiences are becoming so common as to be unremarkable.

# Joe (obesity)

## *The backstory*

There was nothing remarkable about 49-year-old Joe. He worked as an administrator for a company in a large city. But like so many people with a similar income, he lived two hours away in a suburb where he could afford a modest home for his family.

Joe walked to work from the train station (a one-kilometre roundtrip). But he was 170cm tall and weighed 78kg, with a body mass index (BMI) of 27.

In other words, he was overweight. To avoid putting on any more weight he needed to restrict his diet to 1,900 calories per day.

Joe had a bowl of cereal for breakfast, a sandwich for lunch and a home-cooked meal with a glass of wine for dinner.

Those meals alone added up to around 1,900 calories. He also had a coffee with his work colleagues every morning (along with a small muffin), a banana at 2pm and two small biscuits while watching television in the evening.

Those snacks added up to another 500 calories. By the time Joe turned 50 six months later, his BMI was over 30 and he was clinically obese.

While he earned a reasonable living, Joe wasn't inspired by or excited about his work. The family bought a new car the year before, so Joe was tied to a hefty car loan. His wife Bridgette resigned from her nursing job when they conceived their first of three children 10 years ago and hadn't worked for pay since. All three were under 10, with the youngest having asthma. It landed him in the hospital a few times, but since being prescribed a new medication he was much better.

Joe and Bridgette's relationship also had its ups and downs and they often argued about the lack of disposable income.

The couple were committed to doing their best for their boys. Joe would go to a football match on the weekend, but he hadn't participated in any sports since his mid-twenties. Between helping Bridgette with the chores and ferrying the kids to and from sporting clubs, music lessons and birthday parties, there was no time to exercise at a gym or pool.

### The event

Joe rarely visited a doctor. In winter he'd get the occasional chesty cough and make an emergency appointment with whoever was available at the local clinic. But he only did that if Bridgette suggested he might need an antibiotic.

On one particular visit, Joe's doctor checked his blood pressure and told him it was normal. His records included the medical examination he had at 35 for a mortgage application and everything was 'normal' back then as well.

Most of Joe's friends were heavier than him and he still thought of himself as 'healthy.' After all, he walked to work, didn't smoke and had a 'healthy' banana in the afternoon. He also made sure his evening meal was a healthy one.

So, the doctor's comment that he'd put on weight didn't make much of an impression.

### *The outcome*

Joe didn't perceive any risk to his health. He never had time to talk to the doctor about why he enjoyed that coffee and muffin, or the dead-end job he was stuck in because of all the debt. Joe never mentioned his boring job, the tedious household chores, or that the coffee breaks were the highlight of his working week.

Joe's trousers were getting a little bit tighter. Bridgette noticed, but Joe's friends were much bigger than him and he didn't think it worried her. She'd gone up three dress sizes herself since the children were born, so she didn't tease him too much. They had an unspoken agreement not to comment on each other's appearance when there was so much else to worry about. Joe had started wearing extra-large clothes and still thought he looked good. Besides, Bridgette often said she found him attractive.

### The lesson

In most countries it's 'normal' to be overweight, if not obese. It's also normal to live in families and communities where the condition isn't considered 'unhealthy.'

If we want Joe to realise he's on his way to having a chronic illness, we need reframe his condition in a way that compels him to make different lifestyle choices. Public health campaigns can warn Joe he has a problem. But this strategy clearly isn't enough on its own, as the number of people who are overweight and obese continues to spiral upward relentlessly.

The family doctor will only have a few more 15-minute sessions before Joe presents with symptoms of diabetes, cancer or heart disease. Those precious minutes need to be considered carefully as part of a healthcare provider's response to chronic illness.

# Dave (lifestyle)

### The backstory

Dave was 50 and struggling to keep up with the younger men on the soccer pitch. He could still down six pints of beer on Saturday night after the match, but most other nights he was happy to settle for two drinks. Some nights he didn't drink at all.

For the first time in his life, his waist measurement had reached 38 inches (96 cm). He felt too unfit and breathless to do any real exercise. And while he felt well enough, his blood pressure was borderline.

According to his wife, he also snored.

## *The event*

Dave wanted a day off work, so he asked for a medical certificate. He had a headache that morning and didn't think he'd cope at work. As the doctor recorded his blood pressure, Dave mentioned the football team he coached and how he was struggling to keep up with the younger players on the field.

## *The outcome*

Dave was more willing to talk about lifestyle with his doctor than a man half his age who'd come to the clinic with a sprained ankle. He admitted he was concerned about his health and wondered if it wasn't too late to regain his fitness.

## *The lesson*

Dave is one of the one million Australians born between 1962 and 1966, known as Generation X. Having just turned 50, he was now officially 'middle-aged.'

In Australia, people can't access their retirement benefits until they turn 67. Then those benefits may need to last them 20–30 years. Many 50-year-olds still have children at school or college and may even have weddings and accommodations to subsidise.

During people's lives, there are times when the interaction between doctors and patients can be far more positive, especially when it comes to lifestyle modification issues around events such as pregnancy, childbirth, coming of age and retirement.

# Joanna (salt fetish)

## *The backstory*

Joanna is exactly the kind of person healthcare wants to help. An office worker in her forties, Joanna was overweight verging on obese. She lived with her husband and three young children in a modest home, the mortgage consuming a large portion of their combined income.

While she had no symptoms, Joanna was hypertensive and well on her way to long-term illness. She refused to give up salt or deprive herself of junk food. She couldn't see she was at risk. As far as she was concerned, she was 'normal.' Because everyone around her ate the same things, she made no attempt to deal with something she didn't perceive as a real or imminent threat.

## *The event*

When she consulted her doctor just before Christmas, they discussed her diet.

'I like salt, so my food tends to be salty,' she said. 'And most people in my extended family are my size. I thought about reducing my portions, but I like lots of meat. I'm a member at a gym, but I rarely go.'

They talked about her risk of heart disease, and the doctor encouraged her to banish the salt shaker from the table, think again about reducing her portion sizes and make time to go to the gym.

The look she gave her doctor said it all.

'Well, that ain't gonna happen,' she said. 'Besides, it's Christmas. I don't want to be a diet when everyone else is out celebrating.'

## The outcome

Her doctor changed tack and focused on other aspects of her life, including what she did for a living. She became animated for the first time, complaining about the mind-numbing boredom and the lack of appreciation for her efforts. She described it as a 'bullshit job.'

## The lesson

Like many (if not most) people, Joanna was unhappy at work. Anthropologist David Graeber suggests there are millions of people across the world who know they're being paid to do meaningless, unnecessary work. Research suggests this perspective on work can lead to highly destructive behaviours that reduces many people's ability to function in not only their current job, but also any job in the future.

By recognising the roots of Joanna's unhappiness, her doctor can help Joanna reduce her reliance on the income, or even consider getting a better job. But for a strategy like this to work, there must be a focus on the art of doctoring.

Future meetings with Joanna could be opportunities to trigger her when she's motivated and ready to reduce the threat to her health. Because in the end it is only Joanna who can make a difference.

# Frank (snoring)

## *The backstory*

Frank, a 68-year-old part-time office clerk, was on a mix of medications: three different drugs for blood pressure, a statin and two different painkillers.

His problems, as he listed them were fatigue, snoring and back pain.

## *The event*

Frank made a routine appointment for another prescription for his medications.

## *The outcome*

His doctor summarised Frank's problems as obesity, poor diet and a sedentary lifestyle.

'Okay doc,' Frank replied. 'I think I need a referral for my snoring.'

Two weeks previously he wanted a new painkiller. The week before that he asked for a referral to a physiotherapist for his back pain.

## *The lesson*

Frank's doctor needs to forge a long-term relationship with Frank and moderate his expectations about what medicines can do to make him more comfortable. The major challenge will be to persuade Frank he already has the ability to slow or even stop his march towards disability. It seems incredible that someone who can't walk to the end of the street without stopping for breath repeatedly can't see any reason to stop eating junk food or watch television for eight hours a day.

People's bad habits can drive their choices—even when they're aware of their growing disabilities.

# Suzy (alcoholism)

## *The backstory*

Suzy was 52, divorced and unemployed. She was also obese.

Suzy often slept on the street and drank a lot, especially when her social security payments came through. And she was often at the emergency department because she'd hurt herself while she was drunk.

She was destined to become a statistic.

## *The event*

She visited her doctor almost every week. Sometimes she seemed well—especially when she'd had a small windfall of social security payments. But she usually came to complain about her bad luck, ask for support to claim social security or insurance benefits, or get prescriptions for her medication— even though she took it only occasionally.

## *The outcome*

The last time her doctor saw Suzy she was just out of hospital after having yet another alcohol-related accident.

Suzy might be amenable to different choices one day. But her immediate need was someone who would explore and tolerate the complexities of her deeply troubled life. She needed someone who could interpret her cries for help, which were often couched in somatic terms.

### *The lesson*

Suzy was often stigmatised. In recent years, governments worldwide have used the rhetoric of personal responsibility to justify cutbacks in necessary health and social programs. Her doctor made concerted efforts to encourage her to lose weight, drink less alcohol and exercise.

None of them succeeded.

Despite her previous failures, Suzy could turn things around. Or she could be forced to use her social welfare payments for food, in which case she may well have traded food for alcohol. Chances are it wouldn't be a fair trade.

Suzy's responses to life may have been a factor of the negative attitudes she experienced on the street. There's no question her poor choices landed her in trouble. But those who knew her would tell you she wanted something better.

Which is why she deserves her clinician's undivided attention. Disrupting their communication would detract from the chance of her choosing to reinvent herself.

# Angela (night visit)

### *The backstory*

Angela was abused as a child and left home pregnant when she was 16. Six years later, her older partner and only adult companion was violent, especially when drunk. They lived on a meagre income supplemented by welfare payments in a rundown two-bedroom unit miles out of town.

## The event

When Angela called her doctor at 2am one winter morning, it sounded like she was at a party. The music playing in the background was so loud her doctor could barely hear what she was saying.

'My three-year-old son has a fever,' she said. 'He also seems to have a rash and gets upset when I turn the light on.'

'He also says his ear hurts. We have no way of getting to you, doctor.'

Her doctor couldn't be sure what was going on, so he agreed to make a house call.

When the doctor arrived at the house, the allegedly sick three-year-old greeted him at the open door. The child had a mild fever and a runny nose. His parents were in the lounge with a neighbour drinking wine after they'd all enjoyed a takeaway meal. The air reeked of fried chicken and tobacco smoke.

It became clear the child had been unwell since lunchtime the previous day. When he woke up after midnight complaining about a painful ear, his mum decided to get the doctor.

There was no paracetamol (acetaminophen) in the house.

## The outcome

The adults curled up on a sofa with wine and cigarettes obviously thought enjoying themselves was more important than the child's brewing upper respiratory illness.

The doctor took in the scene. A bare lightbulb glowed dimly overhead, revealing a wet sofa surrounded by dirty carpet. Fast food remains littered the floor and a dog was sniffing everyone's heels. The sick child's clothes were filthy and threadbare and a baby was asleep on the sofa. Sitting in the corner was a new TV they'd bought with money they borrowed.

While these people obviously had little money, they could have called for help much sooner than they did. And they could have changed their behaviour in any number of ways.

## *The lesson*

While it seems they'd orchestrated their own misfortune, the whole scene could have been framed very differently. The couple had debts because they borrowed money for the TV and their income rarely lasted a full week.

The doctor didn't see the 'final demand' notices or the threats from money lenders. He didn't notice the bruises on Suzy's torso. He also didn't know about the menial, boring job with its demanding employer.

All of which made it harder for them to be good parents that morning.

Sometimes people can't make better choices for the long term because they already have more problems than they can cope with. The medium and long-term timeframes don't feature in their plans. So, to serve those people, doctors need to be resilient.

# Tegan (cancer)

## *The backstory*

The first time Tegan met her doctor she was 32, single and pregnant. As she approached her baby's due date, she became more and more excited about becoming a mother.

'I want this baby so much,' she said.

## *The event*

After the baby was born Tegan brought her in so her doctor could administer her immunisations. During her second visit she confided that she had a lump in her breast.

'I've had it a few months,' she admitted. 'I think it's because I'm breast feeding.'

The doctor examined the lump in Tegan's breast. It appeared to be benign, but the fact it had persisted for months was a worry. The doctor arranged a mammogram and biopsy and Tegan accepted the referral without hesitation. They both knew this was precautionary, as there were no signs Tegan had breast cancer.

## *The outcome*

The scan and the biopsy were negative and the doctor happily gave Tegan the news during her appointment a couple of weeks later. As Tegan was about to leave she said, 'What I don't understand is this hard lump in my tummy. My partner noticed it the other day when I went to get up off the couch.'

A moment later the doctor confirmed the unmistakable sign of cancer in her liver.

As Tegan was due to see a surgeon about her breast lump anyway, the doctor notified the surgeon about her findings.

Tegan died a week before her daughter's first birthday.

Apparently, Tegan *had* noticed a change in her bowel habit. But she attributed it to her pregnancy and so never mentioned it.

The cancer was in her bowel, not in her breast.

### The lesson

Sometimes even the doctor's best efforts won't save the patient from a bad outcome. In this case, the doctor's goal changed from how to save Tegan's life to how to reduce Tegan's suffering.

# Ryan (poisoning)

### The backstory

The doctor received a call from a worried young girl, who asked him to see her teenage brother who had a sore throat. The doctor didn't think to get any useful information from the youngster and so decided to do a home visit before breakfast.

### The event

The doctor set off before six in the morning. During the drive he realised he'd be working all day (and possibly all night), and then again, the following day at the clinic. He started feeling angry. Why didn't the chap take a couple of cold and flu tablets and call him later, or even come to the clinic later in the morning?

## *The outcome*

The doctor arrived at the house to find an older teenage boy partying with his friends. He was camped out in front of the television with a can of beer in one hand and a cigarette in the other. The house was full of drunk youngsters playing video games.

There were no adults in sight.

The doctor called Ryan into the hallway and produced a flashlight. Ryan insisted his throat was very sore and that nothing was helping. Sure enough, his throat was red and judging by the tender lumps in his neck, infected. He also had a mild temperature.

The doctor wasn't impressed and asked why he didn't just take paracetamol (acetaminophen) and go to bed.

'Well, I didn't want to call you,' he insisted. 'It was my sister who called. Besides, I've taken 20 of those since midnight, and they're not helping.'

Half an hour later he was in the hospital being detoxified from his potentially fatal overdose and being treated for epiglottitis.

If Ryan had done what the doctor was thinking (i.e. take more pills and call for help later in the morning or early afternoon), he may well have died a horrible death from poisoning.

## *The lesson*

As a doctor, you should never make assumptions about patients—even when their behaviour is objectionable.

# Hamish (thief)

## *The backstory*

While making their way home, a medical student and his girlfriend would often stop outside a shop window displaying the crystal paperweight embossed with his university's crest. He dearly wanted to have it. But the price was far more than he could afford.

So, he was thrilled when he opened the Christmas present from his girlfriend and saw the paperweight –a memento of her love.

From that point on it took pride of place on his desk at work.

## *The event*

One day he walked into his office to find the paperweight had disappeared from his desk. He assumed it had been stolen, but so many people had used his office that he couldn't even pinpoint when it was taken, let alone by whom.

One Saturday evening he was called to see Hamish, who was much the worse for wear after his night out. As the doctor began suturing a nasty gash on his forehead, Hamish peered up at him with a cheeky grin and winked.

'You've got one of those paperweights from that university,' he hiccupped. 'So have I.'

## *The outcome*

Hamish couldn't have known his doctor owned such a thing unless he'd been in his office. The doctor realised Hamish had almost certainly stolen his treasured gift.

## The lesson

Sometimes there's no justice in medicine. Just because doctors dedicate their lives to the welfare of their patients doesn't necessarily mean their patients will treat them (or their property) with respect.

The gift was later replaced by the girlfriend who was now his wife and he got to tell this story. He thinks it was worth it.

# Natasha (meningitis)

## The backstory

The doctor's last house call before going home for the day was to the home of six-year-old Natasha. According to the receptionist, she had an earache and was vomiting.

## The event

When the doctor arrived, Natasha's father greeted him like a long-lost relative.

'Thank God you're here,' the father said with a worried look on his face. 'She's in here.'

Natasha was sitting on the couch having clearly just vomited. She had a fever and complained about an earache.

A thorough examination by the doctor found only a red eardrum—an infection that would explain the earache. The doctor prescribed an antibiotic, recommended pain killers and told Natasha's father to take her to emergency if she wasn't better within the next few hours.

The doctor also described possible rashes that couldn't be ignored.

### The outcome

Later that weekend the doctor heard from the local paediatric unit that Natasha *did* develop a rash and now had meningitis but was doing very well. The doctor's initial diagnosis was incorrect and she was a lot sicker than she appeared.

Fortunately, despite the delayed diagnosis Natasha made a complete recovery.

### The lesson

The doctor should have been alerted by the worry etched on the father's face when he arrived. The way people communicate often gives a vital clue when diagnosing health problems. It pays to be alert to these subtle cues.

## Jonathan (tests)

### The backstory

At 27, Jonathan looked fit and healthy. With his regular doctor on holiday, he was given an appointment with another doctor.

### The event

Jonathan began with a clear request.

'I only need one other blood test,' he said to the doctor. 'Doctor Jones organised everything else, but I think I need my vitamin D levels checked.'

There was no need to worry about his vitamin D levels, so they talked more about why he wanted this particular blood test. Jonathan said he hadn't had any blood tests recently and wanted to make sure 'everything was in order before the New Year.'

### The outcome

Sensing Jonathan had anxieties for his health, the doctor started a conversation about them. He discovered that Jonathan knew little about what causes vitamin D deficiency, or that blood tests were no guarantee he wouldn't become vitamin D deficient in the future.

The doctor didn't know why Jonathan's regular doctor had organised the plethora of tests, but something told him there was more to the story.

### The lesson

I can't tell you how this one ends. But what I *can* tell you is this situation is common—especially in health care systems where continuous care is something you can get only by seeing the same doctor.

When organising their health care people don't necessarily make the best choices about who they consult and why. Choice is enshrined in the way the system is organised.

In this case, all the doctor could do is try to understand why it was important for Jonathan to have everything in order before the New Year. There won't always be time.

## Mildred (loneliness)

### The backstory

Mildred was 70 years old and lived alone, with only her small dog for company. She visited her doctor every month.

Her doctor knew she didn't have a lot of money and that sometimes she'd go without her medication because she'd run out of cash. She tried to make ends meet by working as a chef at a greasy spoon. Her boss was a difficult man and often refused to pay what he owed her.

Mildred's doctor had seen her through oesophagitis, osteoporosis, even breast cancer. On each occasion she insisted on waiting for months to be seen as a subsidised patient because she couldn't afford to expedite the investigations.

### The event

One weekend her dog became paralysed and the vet asked for her permission to carry out emergency surgery –a financial commitment she'd be paying off in monthly instalments well into the future.

Her doctor couldn't believe how much she'd agreed to pay.

'That's right Doctor,' she said. 'Two thousand dollars. The vet lets me pay it back in instalments. He did the same a couple of years ago. He's very kind.'

### The outcome

Her dog made a complete recovery, only to die a year later from an unrelated cause. Mildred consoled herself by immediately buying a new puppy.

### The lesson

Sometimes people's choices make no sense in light of the limited information we have about them. If Mildred's doctor hadn't known about her dog, forgoing her own treatment from time to time wouldn't have made any sense.

# Fran (headaches)

## *The backstory*

Fran was somewhere between 35 and 50 years old and always immaculately dressed. When she arrived for her consultations, she was quite cheerful. But the longer they went on, the more morose and dejected she became, cheering up only when she got up to leave.

She was earnest when she first met her doctor.

'I have these terrible headaches,' she complained. 'Nothing has helped so far. But I know *you* can fix it.'

## *The event*

Her doctor set out to find a reason for her chronic headaches. He examined her and performed lots of tests. But when no diagnosis was forthcoming, the doctor ordered a bunch of empirical treatments.

Each time she'd stop taking the prescribed drug for one reason or another—'side effects,' 'the cost of the tablets' or 'inconvenience'—with each excuse more inventive than the last.

Even after visiting several specialists, it became clear that no doctor would ever 'cure' whatever was causing the headaches.

## *The outcome*

The doctor tried a different tack. Recognising she was bored and unhappy, he wondered if dealing with her dysphoria would make her headaches less of an issue. But whatever he suggested, her reply was the same: 'I can't do much with these headaches.'

Oddly enough, she seemed cheerful and able to function perfectly well despite the headaches spanning many years.

## *The lesson*

Who knows why Fran 'needed' a headache that couldn't be treated? But the fact is, some people 'need' their symptoms.

Unfortunately, a doctor's desire to 'cure her' can in fact put her at enormous risk—especially when that doctor is made to believe they're the infamous (but fictional) Dr Gregory House.

Through my training, I learned to be aware of people who were cheerful and could function perfectly well despite their symptoms.

---

Each of these stories offers an important lesson. But they all share a number of elements.

They all involve two 'actors' (the doctor and the patient) who get together on a 'stage' (a house or consultation room) and work through a 'script' (what they say to each other).

What's said is often determined by the persona each 'actor' chooses to adopt. Sometimes 'props' are used to aid the interaction. And finally, there's the 'action' that leads to a particular outcome.

Each element can be considered in its own right. Those who understand this doctor-patient 'play' can sometimes anticipate what's going to happen and influence how it might end.

I call this the Theatre Model©. And I'll be talking more about each element in the chapters that follow.

# 2

# WHY DO PEOPLE SEEK HEALTHCARE?

Before we consider the art of doctoring in any detail, I'd like to offer some context to why healthcare is important in our lives.

In the Organisation for Economic Co-operation and Development (OECD) countries, most adults spend the bulk of their waking hours at work. This environment affects their physical and psychological health and can be both harmful and beneficial. Most of these people will have symptoms of some illness in a given month. Those who seek medical advice typically turn to a family doctor.

So, to achieve good healthcare it's crucial that people get treatment when it's effective and cheap. But providers have adopted convenience and speed as proxies for quality. Healthcare is organised as if most people, such as Suzy who struggles with alcoholism or Fran who complains about persistent headaches, have a temporary and urgent illness. The drive towards speedy services is founded on faith in quick technical fixes.

However, doctors are most effective when they persuade people to make difficult long-lasting changes that protect their wellbeing. Sometimes doctors need to help people tolerate discomfort because no-one has the resources or the ability to cure every conceivable medical problem.

When doctors are encouraged to focus on the funders' priority list of conditions, they may ignore other significant problems that may be affecting the patient's wellbeing. There's a substantial need that isn't being met, and healthcare needs to recalibrate in the same way other businesses focus on serving loyal customers.

Healthcare will fail at every level until doctors deploy their insight to improve how patients like Frank (with his snoring issue) and others feel about visiting a doctor. The best results, especially for Frank, Suzy, Joanna and Joe, would be for people to make better choices. Doctors are well placed to trigger and direct their efforts toward that outcome.

And they do so by practicing the art of doctoring.

---

Before we consider how healthcare can be fixed, we need to revisit the reason people seek help from doctors in the first place. Joe (obesity), Dave (lifestyle) and Joanna (salt fetish) spend most of their waking hours at work. Australians work an average of 34 hours a week, with one in six people working more than 50 hours a week.[6] In contrast, they spend 6–9 hours a week doing housework[7] and almost seven hours a day sleeping.[8]

Similarly, in many parts of the world work is the most important aspect of people's lives:

> *The average working American spends the majority
> of his or her waking hours on the job. Some of us live
> and breathe our work. Others of us work to pay our
> mortgages. Either way, the workplace has become an
> indispensable source of social capital for millions of
> Americans—a center of meaning, membership, and
> mutual support. More than ever, we find our close
> friends and life partners on the job, we serve our
> communities through work-organized programs, and
> we use the office as a forum for democratic deliberation
> with people different from ourselves. Countless studies
> show that a workplace with strong social capital
> enhances workers' lives and improves the employer's
> bottom line.[9]*

Joe's and Joanna's working environments are affecting both their physical and psychological health. Being unhappy at work can increase the risk of long-term illness.

In 2002, approximately 59% of global death was attributable to chronic, non-communicable diseases. That figure is expected to increase to 66% by 2030, and this trend affects people when they decide to retire from work.

A team of researchers found that being forced into early retirement due to illness or poor health can adversely affect an individual's financial security. Furthermore, they have almost as much chance of becoming income poor as those who are unemployed. And of course, it also affects the retiree's family members. By contrast, individuals whose early retirement wasn't associated with poor health fared reasonably well.[10]

A 2009[11] report by the Australian Institute of Health and Welfare outlined the consequences of chronic illness and early retirement on the entire Australian economy. It concluded:

- People with chronic disease averaged 0.48 days off work in the previous fortnight due to their illness, compared with 0.25 days for those without chronic disease.
- The annual loss in workforce participation from chronic disease in Australia was around 537,000 person-years for full-time employees and around 47,000 person-years for part-time employees.
- For full-time employees there was a loss of roughly 367,000 person-years associated with chronic disease, 57,000 person-years in absenteeism related to chronic illness and 113,000 person-years due to death from chronic disease.

And these estimates are *underreporting* the loss in workforce participation. They don't factor in the lower performance of those working while feeling ill, or the unpaid labour force of carers, parents and volunteers.

Given the economic impact of healthcare outcomes, keeping people at work creates significant value. Sick people can't work or retire early. They don't pay taxes.[12] They don't create wealth.

Many people who need healthcare could improve their health outcomes simply by making better choices.

Most people will develop a symptom of some sort in a given month.[13] The minority who seek medical advice will consult a family doctor, while a significant number (such as Joe with his obesity) will seek advice from a non-physician such as a pharmacist. Some (such as Tegan with cancer) will be referred to a hospital by their doctor. Fewer still will be admitted to an intensive care ward like Natasha was for her meningitis.

The key point here is that most people concerned about their health and wellbeing will first seek help in primary care. Their health outcomes will most likely be determined by the care delivered by their family doctor. If Tegan had told her doctor about her bowel symptoms, she might still be alive.

Primary care has the potential to not only constrain healthcare costs, but also have a positive effect on the wellbeing of the taxpaying workforce. When people are distressed, they need doctors to make it easier for them to meet life's challenges.

Unfortunately, clinics tend to operate as if all patients had the same needs. Dave, whose lifestyle choices are affecting his health, has different needs to Pauline who's suffering from pneumonia. Most healthcare systems worldwide are designed as if it doesn't matter which doctor Dave consults or what that doctor knows about his problems. Patients like Pauline are generally expected to make appointments at a time and place that suits the practitioner. They might be seen for less than 15 minutes and leave feeling their questions and concerns weren't addressed.[14] Consequently, both the doctor and the patient can become frustrated. Any of the patients mentioned in the previous chapter may have felt that way given how healthcare is organised.

In recent years, efforts to improve healthcare have focused largely on making doctors more affordable. It's become the proxy metric for quality. Whatever can be measured and quantified is given the highest priority, while everything else that happens in the consulting room that can't be measured is either a distraction or irrelevant.

Commoditising healthcare like this might be convenient for Jonathan, who only wants a blood test. But it doesn't come close to delivering the kind of care that fosters patient empowerment and wellness.

These 'data-driven monitoring for monitoring's sake' consultations can't provide the same standard of care and patient outcomes as a one-on-one consultation with a skilled practitioner who knows Pauline and her circumstances. Joe (obesity) can now visit pharmacists or nurse practitioners, book a video consultation with a doctor he's never met, or use a range of emergency services in hospitals or after-hours primary care centres.

Frank (snoring) can acquire a prescription, referral or sickness certificate with relative ease. He also has easy access to Doctor Google, where he can find any number of dubious treatments. (For example, some people claim that improving wellness is just a matter of paying attention to an increasing list of purported dietetic and hormonal deficiencies.[15])

Along with a slew of new providers and solutions, patients like Fran (headaches) can seek private health alternatives that offer one-to-one bespoke wellness advice. Many people are willing to pay for services and experiences such manicures, hairstyling and acupuncture that helps them 'feel' better but cost more than a visit to a state- or insurance-funded doctor.

At a technical level, the doctor's job is to offer solutions that remove or reduce the threat to a patient's wellbeing. They can do this by studying pathology and therapeutics, which might serve a minority of people well, such as six-year-old Natasha with meningitis and Ryan who almost died from paracetamol (acetaminophen) poisoning. Then, as an acknowledged expert, the doctor can 'educate' the patient or prescribe pills, potions or procedures that alleviate the symptoms and any pain or suffering.

The best outcome is often achieved by helping patients acknowledge and accept that some unpleasant symptoms and minor illness (e.g. the common cold, warts and rashes) are a temporary inconvenience. In this context, appendicitis may seem like a straightforward anatomical malfunction that can be easily fixed with surgery. But the symptoms of a throbbing, inflamed appendix can't be ignored. The patient needs to believe the surgery will relieve the pain and allow them to continue living as before.

Appendectomies, like so many operations, are now relatively minor procedures that have changed beyond all recognition.[16] But what hasn't changed is the persuasion needed to have this invasive but potentially life-saving operation.

We may recognise the importance of doing what's necessary, at least in the context of the potential harm of acting against medical advice. For example, people were misled when they were told a routine vaccine would cause autism in their children.[17]

We must also acknowledge the harm done when people are persuaded to undergo treatment that isn't in their best interests[18], such as the women who experienced more harm than good after agreeing to take long-term hormone replacement therapy.[19]

Doctors operate within a specific political and cultural milieu. They can't act outside the laws of their jurisdiction and can't provide a service to patients if the funder doesn't consider the treatment a 'priority.'

Varicose veins, cataracts and inguinal hernias are good examples of what funders consider 'low priority' conditions. They're not immediately life-threatening and in their early stages may simply be disfiguring or inconvenient.[20] Treatment for these usually involves being put on a waiting list, which means doctors must help patients with these conditions bear the pain and physical limitations until they make it off the waiting list sometime in the future.

So, while doctors need to identify the correct treatment, they also need to overcome resistance to accepting what's in the patient's best interests (or in some cases what serves everyone in a cash-strapped health service). They need to offer comfort, advocacy and reassurance—even when dealing with limited resources.

Chances are the doctor won't have an easy answer for Suzy's alcoholism. But their role is to support and advise, despite the frustrations everyone may experience.

# 3

# THE DOCTOR'S WORLD

In 2014, Devesh Oberoi PhD interviewed men with bowel disease who'd presented late to a specialist and were subsequently diagnosed as having cancer. One of the interviewees suggested the delay might be due in part to a late referral.

'I spoke to my GP that time, and I was concerned about the symptoms. I told him I'd seen some blood on my toilet paper and he said, "Umm, yeah. Since it's fresh blood, it could be piles (haemorrhoids) or something."'[21]

In that particular case the correct diagnosis was made much later and the treatment required was far more invasive. Which is why some experts have called for more research to establish why a cancer diagnosis is sometimes delayed.

While Oberoi was working on his thesis, my research team published secondary data from an experimental study. We reported that a diagnosis of cancer can be missed even when the presentation is straightforward with no distracting issues in the consultation (e.g. other physical illnesses, mental illness or social problems). One in eight 'cases' presented as short video vignettes to doctors in simulations failed to elicit a response that included a referral to a specialist or investigations to establish the diagnosis of cancer.[22]

What's more, when these doctors decided to prescribe something it's doubtful whether the 'patient' would have received any benefit. In some cases that treatment may have even resulted in further harm. When the recommendation was to order tests, the rationale behind ordering some of those tests wasn't immediately apparent. Delays may also have occurred if the test results were negative or misleading.

Numerous audits, including one we published in 2004, established similar patterns. Our 2004 study offered three reasons for failing to recognise patterns of cancer:[23]

- Failure to consider the possibility of cancer as a cause of the symptoms
- Inappropriate or incomplete investigation
- False-negative investigations

Despite this research, some policymakers believe it's appropriate to pay GPs to focus on a specific list of illnesses. Pursuing funded targets distracts doctors from the fundamentals of good doctoring, including giving Mildred (who suffers from loneliness and may consult them about any type of illness) their undivided attention.

When doctors are given an incentive to spend precious time collecting data and ticking boxes, the poor outcomes speak for themselves. We already know results are unsatisfactory in some cases and this should lead to reviewing the direction of policy change when managing doctor performance.[24] In relation to pay for performance (the idea to get the best out of doctors they should be paid for measurable results), the UK's King's Fund concluded in 2010:

> *What evidence does exist suggests that significant*
> *improvements have been made in some areas—*
> *particularly for diseases such as diabetes, heart failure,*
> *and chronic obstructive pulmonary disease—but less*
> *progress has been made for depression, dementia, and*
> *arthritis, and these require a more collaborative care*
> *model for a higher quality of care to be achieved.[25]*

When the incentives for providing 'quality' are financial, they're often limited and introduced piecemeal by redirecting resources from elsewhere in the system. Overall funding for healthcare rarely increases and so what's offered is inadequate at best and often reduces funding in other areas. Healthcare is but one priority for legislators and government agendas are often driven by short-term goals to appease voters and win the next election.

Patients with long-term illnesses have significant unmet needs that affect their quality of life.[26] The future of healthcare depends on adequately serving the needs of those likely to consult a doctor again and again in the coming years. People like Frank (snoring) need to function despite a long-term illness, so they can work and care for others even when they're not at their best.

They also need to believe their doctor understands their perspectives and will always meet their needs. In the business world, such loyalty in a customer is prized. Businesses strive to make customers feel valued. Successful companies are always looking for new ways to delight their customers.

Sadly, in healthcare we often fall short of this goal. We know, but often forget, that what patients crave the most is their doctor's undivided attention. Like a customer in any other business, patients want to feel like they count.

Doctors have both the insight and the wherewithal to redesign the patient experience. We don't have to rely on policymakers to empower us to do better for our patients. If research has taught us anything, it's that the fundamental need in healthcare is for doctors to have superb communication skills.[27] Without that foundation, nothing technology can do for the patient will ever be enough.

Every touch point of the healthcare system should tell a patient, 'We know and care about you.' We may not always be able to cure people. But we can always make them feel like they count. What our patients need as much (if not more) than health targets and cures is doctors who are skilled communicators.

And what we need to do as clinicians is to get back to basics and rediscover the power of the art of doctoring. We need to persuade people like Joe with his obesity and Joanna with her salt fetish to make different lifestyle choices—eat less salt and sugar, drink less alcohol, stop smoking, exercise more. Understanding what drives them to make poor choices, does more to improve their health than trying to fix it when the damage is already done.[28]

Now, let's look at how we can improve healthcare to achieve better results using a back-to-basics approach.

# 4

# THE THEATRE MODEL©

The consultation is where we experience the art of doctoring. It's the meeting between the doctor and the patient, which can result in any outcome. The patient may be guided through the available options, learn how others (and possibly technology) can help and be told who will play a role in their recovery.

How they respond, and whether they act on the information provided, depends on:

- how effectively they both communicate
- whether they have the capacity and the bandwidth to focus on the real problem

In my 30 years as a doctor I've come to appreciate that the consultation is defined by time, place and person. Each element is critical to the successful outcome of that consultation. We need a process that helps us use these three key elements to consistently deliver our best to every patient in every consultation.

A surgeon will wash their hands, gown up, glove up and drape the patient on the operating table before their scalpel goes anywhere near the patient's skin. But when a doctor consults a patient in an office setting there's no such ritual. It can take place in any room with two seats and a desk, as if the staging and choreographing are unimportant.

To try and redesign this way of working, I've developed a process I call 'the Theatre Model©.'

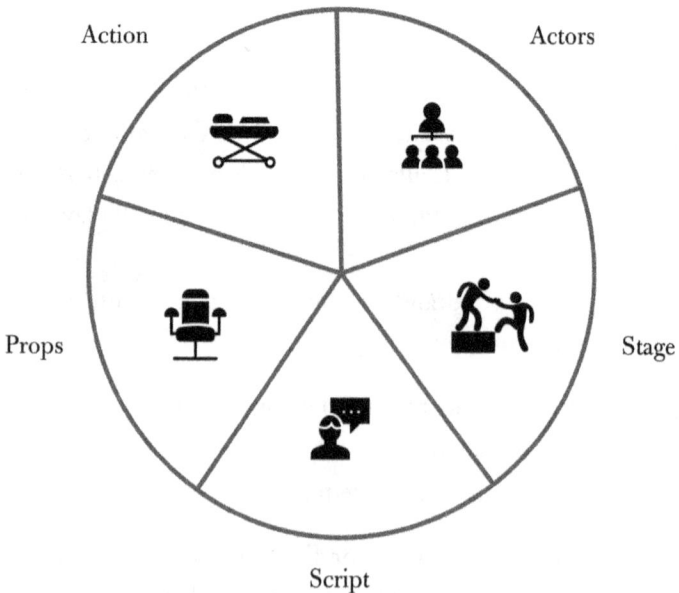

Action

Actors

Props

Stage

Script

**THE THEATRE MODEL©**

This model frames what's seen, heard, smelt, felt and even tasted when patients consult doctors.

The model has five components:

1. **The actors:** the doctor and the patient
2. **The stage:** the building, especially the small room where the actors eventually meet
3. **The script:** what is said
4. **The props:** the tools and other paraphernalia that are part of the consultation
5. **The action:** what is done, including (and especially) the examination

At one time, the place where people met their 'healer' was rich in symbolism. Most of that symbolism has been jettisoned, dumbed down or devalued. People such as Pauline (pneumonia) and Mildred (loneliness) now enter a space devoid of symbolic significance. The person they see may not even be wearing a white coat, much less any other ceremonial garb. They may even enter a virtual space and interact with a 'provider' on screen.

And it's the patient who often pays for this privilege. Their problems are summarised and they're offered an off-the-shelf 'solution' that rarely takes their circumstances (e.g. Pauline having to walk across town to the clinic) into account. The critical transaction is payment, which is done quickly, efficiently and often electronically via a smartphone or tablet. Access and convenience are valued above all else.

This model may work for some patients, such as those with a minor infection (e.g. conjunctivitis) or people like

Jonathan who only want a test to be performed. But it's hopelessly ineffective for patients such as Suzy (alcoholism) who can't succinctly articulate their complex or long-term health problem.

Because a monetary value is attached to the encounter, it could be said that the business model has driven the evolution of the medical consultation. What's rarely considered is that this meeting, aside from any technical considerations, involves issues that are fundamental to our health and wellbeing. When we're sick, tired, distressed or worried, we need to believe in the special qualities of the individual whose attention we seek in that particular place.

As patients, we deeply value anything that promotes intimacy. We're more likely to feel safe and therefore more likely to disclose what's worrying us and why. Elements that help produce that outcome trigger our ability to make better choices on our way to recovery, or at least commit to alternatives that will require effort. We also need these rituals to help us disclose our deepest fears for our wellbeing.

The Holy Grail is cheaper and more effective healthcare. But it starts with the short meeting between doctor and patient. This critical encounter lays the foundations for good healthcare outcomes. Here's a boiled down version of the script, which will be familiar to anyone who has visited a doctor.

> *The patient enters a private room, where an*
> *individual in familiar symbolic garb (perhaps a*
> *white coat or scrubs) deploys equipment seldom seen*
> *elsewhere. This individual (the doctor) can be trusted*

> *to keep secrets and put the patient's interests above*
> *any other consideration. So the doctor is allowed to*
> *hear, see and feel things the patient would otherwise*
> *consider private and confidential.*
>
> *The doctor asks personal questions, which the patient*
> *is expected to answer. The patient can also expect to be*
> *examined and even undress at the doctor's request if*
> *the doctor considers it necessary.*
>
> *The doctor, who is thought to have specialised*
> *knowledge, considers the patient's symptoms and*
> *everything they have seen, heard and felt. The critical*
> *role of the doctor is to alleviate suffering, of which*
> *pain is the most familiar example.*
>
> *The doctor reflects and then offers a remedy, course of*
> *action or note (doctor's certificate).*
>
> *The patient leaves the private room, confident the*
> *personal information they've divulged is safe.*

Sometimes the meeting is related to the obvious effects of disease. Other times the doctor gives the patient a privilege, such as being allowed to be absent from work or having a medical cost subsidised by the state or an insurer.

Occasionally the meeting is to protect society from those who might cause it harm due to mental illness or perhaps the spread of an infectious disease. The solution may involve drugs to improve mental functioning, confinement to a hospital, or one or more vaccines.

Doctors are also explicitly authorised to diagnose and determine a cause of a person's death.

In any case, the consultation is governed by the rules of the community and what is lawful in that jurisdiction. What's legal in some countries (e.g. abortion or euthanasia) may be illegal in others. The decisions made when practicing the art of doctoring are crucial because they govern the prognosis, whether it's relieving distress, improving if not ending symptoms, circumventing decline or preventing death.

## The actors

A theatrical scene is meaningless if we don't know about the characters. In medicine we rarely consider this aspect of the encounter, as if it makes little difference to the outcome unless it can be summarised as a number.

Every consultation has two actors: the doctor and the patient. Each will assume a distinct persona, which may well be different to the other personas they assume in their day-to-day lives. Having said that, the doctor is likely to take the same approach to consults with every patient and every patient is likely to respond in a characteristic way.[29]

The doctor's greeting style is likely to be consistent from case to case. Some will greet their patient formally, while others won't even offer to shake their hand. They'll be called either by their first name or their last name. While some doctors make lots of eye contact, others rarely shift their gaze from their desk, computer or equipment.

Some doctors will disclose a lot about themselves—their partners, families, pets or holidays. Others will rarely talk about their private lives. Some will make jokes, while others will be serious, if not forbidding. Some doctors will be emotional in their responses. Some will be inscrutable.

Each patient will also present themselves differently. For example, Suzy (alcoholism) will come across very differently to Tegan (cancer) and Dave (lifestyle). Like Jonathan (tests), some will be very matter of fact and come with a specific list of needs and wants. Patients like Joanna (salt fetish) will be reluctant to share the reason for their visit until they feel they have a connection with the doctor.

Some will readily disclose a great deal about their circumstances, ideas, concerns or expectations. Some will convey little or nothing. Some patients will be fluent communicators, while others will struggle to make themselves understood due to linguistic, cultural, psychological or physical limitations.

Most patients will be of the same ethnicity as their doctor but sometimes they'll have very different backgrounds or financial circumstances. It's unusual for doctors to know much about patients they don't see regularly that isn't documented in their medical records. A doctor may be able to cite the patient's blood pressure but know nothing about their home life or occupation.

## The stage

The consultation usually takes place in a small room—a private space designed for no more than two or three people. It sometimes smells of disinfectant or air freshener and the walls may be decorated with posters or leaflets. Certificates, awards and photos of the doctor's family may be on display. The room may contain basic furniture—seats, a desk, an examination table. In many countries I've worked in the doctor occupies the largest chair, often a tall-backed leather office seat placed close to a desk. In other countries the doctor's seat may not be the largest but will have other details that differentiate it from the others.

This room is the doctor's 'stage.'

Healthcare organisations rarely think about setting that stage to achieve the best outcome for patients. But on every other 'stage' where one actor hopes to influence another (such as retail environments), these details are crucial.

Joanna (salt fetish) and Joe (obesity) need to be convinced to change their lifestyle. That already difficult task is made even harder when it takes place in a setting that looks like an airport terminal.

## The script

In every consultation there's a 'script'—what one person says and how the other person responds. Often the words spoken by one actor are deliberately chosen to elicit a specific response from the other.

In similar circumstances the doctor will often say the same thing, explain symptoms the same way and offer treatment choices using the same words, all in a set sequence. The way the doctor greets the patient, the words they use and the way they deliver them all set the tone of the consultation.

Similarly, the patient may choose to convey their problems in specific terms to elicit a particular outcome. A symptom may be framed as a 'severe' cough or the 'worst ever' headache, conveying the expectation that only a prescription treatment will solve the problem.

Much of the language is coded and repeated between the same set of doctors and patients. What's said, how it's said and the order the information is given affects the outcome of the consultation. Suzy (alcoholism) most likely described her symptoms in a particular way because she needed the doctor to believe she'd take their advice, follow their instructions, complete the course of pills or follow through with the specialist appointment.

## The props

The clothes doctors wear and the props they use during the consultation can affect how patients perceive them. These perceptions can affect whether the patient is open to the advice or treatment the doctor prescribes.

Every doctor has their own style. Some might don a white coat or theatre scrubs. Some might wear a suit and tie. Some will dress less formally, or even casually. How they dress often reflects their attitudes toward the consult. The dress code may be a proxy for a more relaxed approach or indicate a formality and barrier that delineates personal boundaries when sharing information, prescribing treatments or ordering tests.

The other props in the room are the instruments on display or used to examine the patient. These have symbolic significance in the consultation. In particular, the stethoscope, reflex hammer and auroscope (used to examine the ear) are classic instruments associated with the healing power of medicine.

How these instruments are displayed and used will influence how patients feel about the consultation and indeed whether they trust the doctor's advice. Every patient I described in Chapter 1 would have reacted to what they saw, felt, heard, smelled and even tasted at the clinic.

## The action

What the doctor and patient do during the course of the consultation is the 'action.' Their body language, level of eye contact and position relative to each other all change how the patient will feel and respond.

The doctor can influence the outcome by where they choose to sit. Sitting at a desk or in a special chair may emphasise their authority during the consult, while sitting beside the patient or at the edge of a desk can convey a feeling of partnership. Making eye contact with the patient implies the doctor is interested in what's being said, but breaking eye contact at critical junctures can suggest they're not interested or even engaged in the patient's story, invalidating what the patient is trying to say.

The examination is a crucial part of the action. Seeing a doctor is one of the few occasions when intimate physical contact between strangers is permitted. The doctor may need to touch parts of the patient's body that are normally hidden under layers of clothing such as their chest, their abdomen and their private parts. Patients may feel dissatisfied (at the very least) if they're not examined. The doctor also risks a diagnostic failure and a subsequent medicolegal complaint.

The examination itself may be part of the therapy offered. Examining the patient is about building trust with them. Pauline and Mick (pneumonia) and perhaps Frank (snoring) would have been dissatisfied at not being examined, even if the advice offered later was questionable.

The action concludes with the elements that mark the end of the consultation. This can include signing documents to approve special medicines or tests which the patient may have expected to receive. Some doctors are liberal in their use of tests and drugs. Some will routinely refer patients to other health practitioners, while others will be less inclined (if not reticent) to do so. Some doctors will regularly prescribe antibiotics, tablets to induce sleep, antidepressants and medicines to promote weight loss. Others will do so much less often, if at all.

Having undue faith in these practices can lead to them being seen as a proxy to improving outcomes. Prescribing a drug or test means the doctor is actually 'doing something,' and the other elements of the encounter should be either taken for granted or considered to have no real value.

In an era where convenience and value for money are on the same side of the equation, the patient's problems and technological 'quick fixes' are framed within the same small window. The broader picture—why the patient is visiting the doctor, the way they present their problems and how the doctor diagnoses them—is ignored. This liberal approach to drugs and surgical procedures may account for the growing incidence of costly medical mistakes reported in the popular press and medical literature.[30]

Healthcare improvements often fail because it's assumed all that's needed is to give the provider an incentive. To those trying to improve it, a hernia repair (arguably a technical fix) is no different to advising people how to manage their weight (Joe), navigate depression or tackle an addiction (Suzy).

Framing the consultation as theatre allows us to consider each component of this uniquely human experience and how it can be refined to include what we've learned from behavioural economists, medical sociologists, designers and psychologists. This structure can bring us back to the essence of the art of doctoring.

In Part 2 we'll be looking at the patient and doctor roles within the context of epidemiological, social, economic and cultural changes over the past three decades. Many healthcare critics assume the measurable outcomes of the consultation— ordering tests and prescribing drugs—are the most important element of the encounter. However, the first and possibly most accomplished doctor, Imhotep of Egypt, never prescribed an antibiotic or ordered an X-ray.[31] The role of the 'medicine man' is and always was socially ordained. As the late Professor James McCormick from Trinity College Dublin put it, the doctor is a 'father figure, not a plumber.'[32]

The challenge when considering the elements of the Theatre Model© individually is that it's difficult to tease out their importance without referencing the other elements. Therefore, the stage (clinic or room) matters because of its effect on:

- the actors (doctor or patient)
- what is said (script)
- the influence of the props (what's on display and deployed in that space)

- what happens in that space (the action and how it's explained to the patient)

The art of doctoring combines all of these elements to create a unique and powerful experience. We must pay particular attention to each element, as they can all influence both the patient and the doctor.

# 5

# THE PATIENT
## *(Actor 1)*

This chapter focuses on a key participant in the art of doctoring—the patient.

In OECD countries, people such as Frank (snoring) and Pauline (pneumonia) are getting older and sicker. Risk factors for lifestyle-related, long-term illnesses are becoming increasingly common. Most people consult a family doctor at least once a year and usually more often. Social norms see people seeking medical advice sooner rather than later. People steadily gain weight, becoming overweight or obese by middle age. Suzy (alcoholism) continues to risk her wellbeing for various complex reasons, including commercial interests that promote and profit from her bad choices. While the dangers of junk food and alcohol is publicly acknowledged, Suzy and others like her continue to make bad decisions.

Doctors are given the opportunity to influence Joe (obesity) in a few teachable moments when they can appeal to his heart as well as his mind. These opportunities are unique to each patient, but all involve knowing why the patient is visiting that specific doctor at that specific time.

Dave's attitude to his occupation and the time of year may both be significant factors, particularly when it comes to eating too much. Poverty and boredom can promote harmful habits because they reduce people's ability to cope with problems in a positive way. When considering why people such as Mildred don't invest in their health, people rarely consider the health benefits of pet ownership, which is becoming increasingly common. Then there are commercial interests that promote 'effortless' solutions rather than tackling the underlying cause of the problems, which may well be the person's poor choices.

We also need to understand that not every patient has a disease. These days doctors have other roles (e.g. custodians of national or insurance company resources) and so they often see patients who don't need prescribed medicines or have issues that can only be resolved with drugs or a scalpel.

The developed world has an ageing demographic.[33] More than half the population in most OECD countries is now more than 35 years old.[34] Accordingly, the proportion of people with risk factors for long-term illness is rising, especially as sedentary lifestyles and overconsumption significantly affect their wellbeing.[35]

When I was at medical school in the 1980s, 10% of Australia's population was obese. By 2015 this proportion tripled to 30%. Sixty percent of Australians are currently overweight (if not technically obese) and that figure is rapidly approaching eighty percent.

Most middle-aged people are either already sick or have risk factors for significant diseases that will manifest sooner or later. Public health experts have been predicting this rising tide of lifestyle-related conditions for at least half a century.[36]

Another accepted statistic is that 80% of people will develop symptoms of some sort in a 30-day period.[37] Fewer than half of these will consider seeing a doctor and those who do will usually see a family doctor. Yet 80% of people will see a family doctor every year because not everyone who comes to the clinic is there because they feel sick.[38]

People such as Suzy (alcoholism), Mildred (loneliness) and Pauline (pneumonia) are generally offered short appointments, despite epidemiological trends showing they have multiple and complex problems that need more time to unpack.

The number of consultations per person per year is also increasing. In Australia, those who see doctors are likely to do so five times a year on average. People such as Frank (snoring) and Mildred (loneliness) are an established and loyal clientele whose growing needs are anticipated. Yet the system remains configured much as it was in the 1980s and perhaps even earlier.

## *The New Normal*

For most people it is now normal:

- To fit into extra-large clothes sizes[39]
- To have large portion sizes when they dine out
- For everyone over the age of 14 to consume alcohol on a weekly[40] basis
- For teenagers to acquire alcohol mainly from friends or acquaintances (45.4%) or from parents (29.3%)[41]
- To have used cannabis one or more times (33% of all people over 14)[42]
- To drink and drive (more than 10% of people)[43]

- To lose their virginity before the age of 16 (i.e. before the age of consent) and have multiple sex partners[44]
- To access pornography at least once a month (66% of all men and 41% of all women), making about half of internet traffic sex-related[45]
- To join a gym but never attend[46]
- To spend more than five hours a day on a smartphone[47]
- To eat food containing too much salt[48]

The problem isn't a lack of public awareness. A 2018 poll found that:

- 78% of Australians believe Australia has a problem with alcohol consumption
- 74% believe those drinking habits would worsen over the next five to ten years
- 81% a growing majority believe more should be done to reduce alcohol-related harm[49]

Despite this awareness, the problem continues to grow unabated. Tobacco and alcohol consumption are continually promoted in the media[50] (particularly social media[51]). But a 10% price increase on alcohol reduced consumption by an average of only 5%.[52] Similarly, every 10% increase in the price of tobacco reduces consumption by about 4%.[53]

At a public health level, the effect of doctors 'advising' people to attend to their lifestyle is very modest because of the powerful and ubiquitous drivers of poor choices fuelled by those who profit from them. Which is why:

- 1,700 new cases of dementia are reported in Australia each week. This condition is linked to poor lifestyle choices and affects one person every six minutes or so.[54]

- Cardiovascular disease affects one in six Australians.[55]

- In 2014/15, 34% of Australians aged 18 years and over had high blood pressure or were prescribed medication and yet 68% of those weren't taking any medication.[56]

- One in two Australian men and one in three Australian women will be diagnosed with some sort of cancer by age 85.[57]

Joe is at risk of becoming a statistic in the 'globesity' epidemic.[58] All that protects him is the ingenuity and interest of those who care enough to help him turn things around. To improve Joe's health outcomes, we need to trigger his efforts at making different choices when he's motivated and has a clear path to achieving his goals.

There's no better opportunity than during a visit to the doctor.

All evidence suggests that if health communication was more effective, we could achieve many of our collective healthcare service goals. We need to define the ideal consultation outcome, because the metrics we've used so far haven't managed to reflect the needs of both doctors and patients.

From Joe's perspective, this means having an experience that effectively engages him to make choices that protect his wellbeing. From his doctor's perspective, it means work that's fulfilling, rewarding and sustainable.

The consultation needs to add value to the lives of both people involved. The health professional needs to be rewarded and the patient needs to feel the consultation was worth the price—subsidised or otherwise.

In response to the significant challenges in healthcare (particularly chronic and complex diseases) it's easy to blame doctors for not successfully engaging with their patients. For example, we could blame:

- Joe's doctor for not getting him to make better choices and develops better habits
- Suzy's doctor for not getting her to control her excessive drinking
- Joanna's doctor for not getting to reduce her salt consumption and take better care of herself

You might be thinking, "If only doctors would do their job and tell these people to eat and drink less, exercise more, take a break from electronic devices and slow down when driving cars." Companies can profit from Joe's bad choices and will therefore promote such habits (directly or indirectly) for their own commercial gains. Consumers are affected by many factors, including:

- their genes
- their families
- their communities
- their friends and colleagues
- their culture
- the media

- their education
- their lived experience
- their geography

This idea is captured in Bronfenbrenner's Ecological Model:[59]

> *At the core of Bronfenbrenner's ecological model is the child's biological and psychological makeup, based on individual and genetic developmental history. This makeup continues to be affected and modified by the child's immediate physical and social environment (microsystem) as well as interactions among the systems within the environment (mesosystems). Other broader social, political and economic conditions (exosystem) influence the structure and availability of microsystems and the manner in which they affect the child. Finally, social, political, and economic conditions are themselves influenced by the general beliefs and attitudes (macrosystems) shared by members of t he society.[60]*

Poor-quality food is cheap and readily available to people like Joe (obesity) and Joanna (salt fetish). They've been seeing and hearing about it in advertisements since childhood.[61] On the other hand, fresh fruit and vegetables are less accessible, more expensive and of varying quality in most countries.[62]

Areas with fewer food choices are also among our most economically disadvantaged. Residents generally have less disposable income to spend on healthier food options. In some places, diets consist mainly of food with little nutritional value.

The revenues of fast food companies provide startling evidence on the profitability of catering to poor eating habits. One report indicates that a multinational fast food company paid $500 million in taxes to the Australian government and might be due to pay more.[63]

Joe (obesity) spends more time at work than almost anywhere else. Expressed in terms of a percentage of life, a 39.2-hour work week (39 hours and 12 minutes) is equivalent to:

- 14% of a person's total life over the course of 76 years (the average predicted lifespan for people born in the year 2000 according to the Office for National Statistic's National Life Tables for the United Kingdom).
- 23.3% of their total time during the course of a 50-year working life.
- 21% of their total waking hours over a 76-year lifespan, assuming eight hours of sleep a night.
- 35% of their total waking hours over a 50-year working life, assuming eight hours of sleep a night.
- 50% of their total waking hours during any given working day.[64]

That's a significant chunk of Joe's life. But like Joe, many people around the world are disengaged at work—a variable associated with other problematic behaviours. As Faragher and colleagues reported in the *British Medical Journal*:

*A systematic review and meta-analysis of 485 studies with a combined sample size of 267,995 individuals were conducted, evaluating the research evidence linking self-report measures of job satisfaction to measures of physical and mental wellbeing. The overall correlation combined across all health measures was r=0.312 (0.370 after Schmidt–Hunter adjustment). Job satisfaction was most strongly associated with mental/psychological problems; strongest relationships were found for burnout (corrected r=0.478), self-esteem (r=0.429), depression (r=0.428), and anxiety (r=0.420). The correlation with subjective physical illness was more modest (r=0.287).[65]*

There's also increasing evidence linking job dissatisfaction to the most significant health challenge we face which is obesity. A survey of nurses in Ohio concluded that, "Disordered eating differed significantly based on perceived job stress and perceived body satisfaction. Nurses with high levels of perceived job stress and low levels of body satisfaction had higher disordered eating involvement."[66] More recently, research reported that obesity rates varied across industries and between races employed in different sectors.

*Obesity trends differed substantially overall as well as within and between race-gender groups across employment industries. These findings demonstrate the need for further investigation of racial and sociocultural disparities in the work-obesity relationship to employ strategies designed to address these disparities while improving health among all US workers.[67]*

Experts suggested a possible explanation for these trends.

> *125 participants from 5 Chinese information technology companies…showed that when participants experienced higher levels of job demands in the morning, they consumed more types of unhealthy food and fewer types of healthy food in the evening. Besides, sleep quality from the previous night buffered the effect of morning job demands on evening unhealthy food consumption. Study 2 used data from 110 customer service employees from a Chinese telecommunications company and further demonstrated a positive association between morning customer mistreatment and evening overeating behaviours, as well as the buffering effect of s leep quality.[68]*

Given this data, doctors can ask Joe a useful question: "What do you do for a living and how do you feel about it?" Consider what people choose to eat while they work or during breaks. Snacks have become the fourth meal of the day— accounting for 580 extra calories daily, mostly from beverages—and may be a primary contributor to the obesity problem.[69]

## Teachable moments

Doctors can make a difference to those who see themselves at risk of harm through a 'teachable moment'. During these moments, patients such as our snorer Frank could be triggered to make better choices. To create these moments the encounter between the doctor and the patient needs to be staged and choreographed to maximise the human connection.

Evidence shows that regardless of how they consult patients, doctors often don't know the context of their patients' problems.[70] Frank's doctor probably doesn't know much about his partner, working conditions, debts, home life or health literacy. Yet the health service still expects doctors to address risk factors for physical pathology and psychopathology effectively, which in Frank's case means delaying (if not stopping) his slide towards long-term illness.

It's important to know how patients are experiencing other aspects of their lives. Successful services and products make people feel they have a choice and that they're in charge. The 'best' ones make people think buying the product or service was a smart move because it allows them to do what they want to do. When money changes hands, there's an expectation that the buyer will feel good about their purchase and walk away convinced it was worth the money. If they don't, then chances are the product won't be around for very long.

That 'smart move' feeling is important when Suzy (alcoholism) or Fran (headache) estimate the value of whatever they've purchased. Of course, the feeling is most noticeable in medicine when prompt action saves a life. It was certainly true for Ryan (poisoning) and Natasha (meningitis) and may well have been for Tegan (cancer) as well.

These occasions are rare, especially in family medicine. Even when patients have symptoms, they often have (or are assumed to have) a self-limiting illness that doesn't require prescribed drugs. Treating the symptoms would provide little if any relief and could even do harm.

When obesity isn't recognised as a problem, we lose the opportunity to impress Joe (obesity) about its importance—especially when compared to more dramatic and heroic efforts such as saving Natasha (meningitis).

Which means primary healthcare needs to do more to become a 'lovemark.'[71]

Saatchi & Saatchi CEO Kevin Roberts suggests the key ingredients for creating lovemarks are:

- **mystery:** great stories: past, present and future; taps into dreams, myths and icons; and inspiration
- **sensuality:** sound, sight, smell, touch, and taste
- **intimacy:** commitment, empathy, and passion

A lovemark delivers beyond a person's expectations of great performance. It reaches their hearts as well as their minds, creating an intimate, emotional connection that people don't imagine themselves living without.[72]

Medicine has enough equity to become one.

A 50-year-old person may have parents in their 70s and 80s. If so, they'll see their parents getting older and sicker and perhaps harbour worries about their health and long-term care expenses. This can prompt significant self-reflection.

> It is in their 50s, for example, that most people first think of their lives in terms of how much time is left rather than how much has passed. This decade more than any other brings a major reappraisal of the direction one's life has taken, of priorities, and, most notably, how best to use the years that remain.[73]

By the time people turn 50:

- most are overweight or obese
- their risk of hypertension begins to rise
- some men experience impotence and women become menopausal[74]
- many start wearing reading glasses[75]
- the prevalence of hearing loss increases substantially[76]

Fifty-year-olds need to stay healthy because in most OECD countries early retirement isn't an option. Within this context, Dave and his doctor focused more generally on his physical wellbeing. This 'teachable moment' allowed them to discuss some simple strategies: reducing portion size, drinking less, committing to more exercise and keeping an eye on his blood pressure.[77]

More than ever before, Dave was eager to invest in his health and change his lifestyle. Which was good, because at his age only one in 15 men have heart disease. As a 60-year-old, the ratio would be one in four.[78]

For Dave, now is the time to invest.

Being in Australia, Dave's doctor is probably also in his 50s.[79] This doctor will reflect the population mean with regard to their body shape. Evidence suggests that to make the consultation with people like Dave more effective, doctors must address their own expanding waistlines.[80] No policy change or grant is needed to forge the connection. Doctors simply need to recognise and enhance the effect of what they're trained to do.

The average body mass index (BMI) of Western males in their 40s is between 25.6 and 28.4.[81] The numbers are similar for Western women.[82]

In other words, most of them are overweight.

In most OECD countries, people don't gain weight steadily through the year. Instead they tend to overeat from the end of November until mid-January. With seemingly endless opportunities to consume sugary treats, most people add a kilo to their already growing girth. Research shows that during the end-of-year holiday season, adults consistently gain 0.4 to 0.9 kg.[83]

Within the theatre of the consultation, doctors and other healthcare professionals need to be able to raise the issue of overindulgence without putting a damper on the festivities.

Nothing is more evident in public health statistics than the role health behaviours play in accidents, illness and disease.[84] In a published series of studies, Lester Breslow and his colleagues revealed that men who successfully followed seven health habits had lower morbidity and mortality rates than those who followed six. Those who followed six of the habits had better health than those who followed five and so on.[85]

Kayman, Bruvold and Stern demonstrated that people who develop their own diet and exercise plans are more successful at achieving and maintaining weight loss than those who play a more passive role.[86] Each year, millions of people successfully quit the smoking habit (usually after several attempts) and most who quit do so on their own.[87]

Individuals such as Suzy have a fundamental right to choose their own lifestyle. Some would argue that with this right comes the responsibility to make wise choices. This is the most compelling reason to target individuals with innovative solutions.

The outcome of Breslow's work is that given the right information, people will make the right choices. Suzy knows that when she drinks too much, she's likely to injure herself. She also knows she's at significant risk for cardiovascular disease and that her poor diet is contributing to her problems. She had bariatric surgery but didn't like the restrictions it imposed on her binging and had the surgery reversed.

Knowing is not enough.

One point of view redefines being ill as being guilty.[88] As epidemiologists such as S. Leonard Syme have pointed out, people at progressively lower socioeconomic status (SES) levels have correspondingly fewer opportunities to control the circumstances and events that affect their lives.[89] Conversely, for individuals at higher SES levels, higher income and greater discretion, latitude and control over their lives may contribute to a more generalised sense of 'control over destiny,' which in turn may enhance their health behaviours and outcomes.

In their 2013 book *Scarcity*, Mullainathan and Shafir postulated that people who lack something can't be expected to behave 'rationally'[90] (i.e. doing what professionals, or society for that matter, might consider necessary for their own good). But Suzy (alcoholism) and Angela (home visit) are perfectly rational in the sense that they behaved in ways consistent with having to live with 'scarcity' (i.e. where the lack of something poses an imminent threat that warrants an immediate fix).

For Suzy that means either dealing with the debt notices, the need to eat and the craving for alcohol, or doing what she knows will make her feel better temporarily: having a drink, filling a shopping basket or eating a cheap burger and chips.

For Angela it meant waiting until she could give her child her full attention, then deciding she didn't really know what was best for the child and summoning a doctor in the middle of the night.

What's challenging is that some people who have already developed a potentially life-limiting illness can't be 'educated' to make different choices if they can't admit even how and why they're contributing to their own demise.

For healthcare to actively promote wellbeing, we need to find ways to help people identify when they're bored (for example) instead of just focusing on the health consequences. The role of doctors needs to include tackling harmful habits and not be limited to therapeutics.

Also, the extent to which patients are willing to seek help can influence the efforts doctors make to deal with the issue's patients bring to their attention. A few years ago, our team audited a number of doctors' clinics with marked discrepancies in the number of drugs prescribed to reduce high blood pressure in older people. The team (which included the doctors who prescribed the drugs) concluded that patients concerned about their high blood pressure were more likely to receive active treatment than those who were less concerned.[91]

There may be many reasons for this, but boredom may be one worth considering.

> *Our culture's obsession with external sources of*
> *entertainment—TV, movies, the Internet, video*
> *games—may also play a role in increasing boredom. "I*

> *think there is something about our modern experience*
> *of sensory overload where there is not the chance*
> *and ability to figure out what your interests, what*
> *your passions are," says John Eastwood, a clinical*
> *psychologist at York University in Toronto.*[92]

There's no pill for an unhappy life.

The demand for primary care continues to rise. It's tempting to assume the drivers for this trend are the same as always: infections, gluttony, sloth, ageing, substance abuse, accidents and genetics. Yet apart from the literature records, practitioners know very little about Frank and Mildred's biographies.

So, what does family medicine actually do and what does this tell us about the way forward?

If family medicine needs to be reformed, we first need to recognise its limitations. For people who are living:

- in relative poverty
- with multimorbidity
- with competing priorities in complex lives

we can no longer respond to their degenerative and chronic conditions with more of the same primary care.

A family doctor can't 'cure' Suzy's divorce, child abuse, boredom, debts, loneliness, poor parenting, illiteracy, bad housing, noisy neighbours or unsafe neighbourhood. Seeing a family doctor for 10 or 15 minutes won't change her circumstances, no matter how frequently she visits.

Perhaps a perceived failure to improve Suzy's health outcomes is driving healthcare reform. At best her doctor might help her cope. At worst, he could add to her problems by prescribing treatments that make her sick.

It's also possible that some of her symptoms (which so far have been linked to her stress) actually have a biological basis and so trying to deal with the symptoms alone could be misguided. After all, such thinking led to the discovery that a bacterium causes stomach ulcers and not stress or spicy food.[93] I doubt a bacterium is causing *all* of Suzy's symptoms, but it may be causing some of them.

### *The other 'person' in the consultation*

We have one of the highest rates of pet ownership in the world. Thirty-nine percent of Australian households have a dog. 50% of Australians share their household with at least one cat and/or dog,[94] compared to only 35% sharing their household with a child under 16. As a result, our pet care industry is worth an estimated $8 billion annually.

Companionship is the driving reason behind pet ownership. Australians shower their pets with gourmet food, protect them with insurance and pamper them with reflexology, acupuncture and hydrotherapy. Pet food has been compared to baby food in terms of resilient market performance. Most supermarket chains have at least half an aisle now stocking chilled pet food. As journalist Julie Power wrote, "Most pet owners consider their pets to be members of the family and this has a powerful impact on how and what people buy."[95]

This trend has taken medicine by surprise.

It may be prudent to ask if the patient has a pet and whether that pet is well. This is especially the case for pensioners such as Mildred, whose dog or cat may be the only companion they have. The impact of pet ownership on health continues to be debated. While it's considered beneficial for reasons that aren't entirely clear,[96] being responsible for a pet may negate all the benefits. Worrying about the dog barking and annoying neighbours or damaging property can be stressful.[97]

Healthcare practitioners might ponder the effect these surrogate family members have on the lives of people such as Mildred. For some people and pensioners in particular, 'high levels of grief may also be experienced in the event of a pet's death. Other aspects include cost, time and behavioural problems that may lead to further stress, anxiety and loneliness.'[98]

Doctors don't think twice about asking a patient whether they smoke or drink alcohol, or to reveal more intimate details. But they rarely ask whether the patient has a pet. This might explain a lot, especially in a world where it's 'normal' for many people to be unhappy at work, overweight, reliant on alcohol, bored, lonely and living with both a chronic illness and an expensive pet.

These 'normal' people are also subject to magazine and internet advertisements suggesting that all they need to 'fix' their unhappy life is a valid credit card.

We've all seen ads that start with "Are you fed up with/ suffering from" followed by one of the following:

- weight gain?
- feeling tired, especially at 3pm?
- feeling foggy?
- waking through the night?

- unable to remember things?
- depression and irritability?
- having no interest in sex?
- constipation?
- aching muscles and joint pain?
- muscle cramps?
- worrying you may be infertile?
- craving sugar and carbs?
- feeling the cold?
- hair loss?
- using coffee and alcohol to lift yourself up?

According to the advertisers, the problem is probably a hormonal deficiency, food allergy or dietary issue, which can be solved quickly and easily by purchasing their product. According to them, Frank (snoring) doesn't need to exercise more, change his eating habits, drink less alcohol, find a more suitable job or improve his relationships. Yet we know from a plethora of research that Frank's expectations can drive better outcomes, even when the active ingredient is a placebo.[99]

## *Not sick*

The demand for appointments in general practice is much the same, regardless of payment structures. People need to see a doctor for a variety of reasons—usually to get a diagnosis, but sometimes just to get the doctor's signature (as was the case with Dave).

One reason is to certify that they are 'sick,' in doing so grant them the 'sick role'—a term used in medical sociology regarding sickness and the rights and obligations of the affected.[100] (Fran may have visited her doctor for the same reason.)

By assuming the sick role, an individual is legally and socially exempted from work. They'll be expected to rest, take medication, be confined to a home or hospital and/or attend a clinic. For those involved in accidents or who have a life-limiting illness or infection, this is reasonable. But sometimes the reason for needing a certificate isn't so clear-cut. Employers can demand that someone taking time off to deal with a cold or family crisis, or to care for a sick child have the episode certified by a doctor.

This adds to the demand for appointments.

Some countries (e.g. the UK) have introduced legislation that entitles people to take short breaks for these reasons without having to produce a medical certificate (doctor's note).[101] However, employers or supervisors can still force their staff to obtain the requisite note or stand accused of malingering. So, people often turn up to primary care clinics with a minor illness that doesn't require a doctor's intervention.

The problem isn't the illness, but rather the employer's reaction to people needing time off to cope with life. They assume anyone can function normally with a minor illness, regardless of what else is going on in their life. A cold can be hard to bear when someone is in an unhappy relationship, bored, depressed or anxious.

The other reason people need a doctor's appointment is to complete a medical examination for insurance and fitness to drive purposes. That might be the case for Mick, who may think he needs to keep his driver's license now that his wife Pauline is so sick, despite his frailty. His doctor might spend a significant amount of time on such administrative chores.

The doctor will also need to write letters and fill in forms, whether it's to make a referral, secure a payment or for legal purposes. While not part of the doctor's primary role, the clinic's design and function seem more attuned to these tasks than to seeing people who want attention because they feel unwell.

What about the doctors? What effect do they have on the theatrical meetings between doctor and patient? It's long been recognised that the doctor is a potent factor in therapy. Michael Balint, the father of modern-day general practice, coined the phrase 'drug doctor' to emphasise the impact doctors can have on their patients' response and recovery from illness.[102] Clearly the doctor is one of the actors but they're also a prop in so far as they have a symbolic significance and are therapeutic in the art of doctoring.

# 6

# THE DOCTOR
## *(Actor 2)*

Those privileged enough to practice the art of doctoring compete with others to enter medical school. After graduating they need to study and sit exams for years before they can finally enter the speciality of their choice.

One way to maintain an effective medical workforce might be to increase doctors' resilience and professionalism, starting from when they're still medical students. Despite training more doctors than ever before, there's a shortage of clinicians willing to serve the patients I've talked about in the poorest parts of any country or in specialties that pay comparatively little.

Some junior doctors may struggle to find jobs. Many will never work in what they once considered a lucrative and prestigious specialty at a location of their choosing.

Doctors can also be influenced by psychological stress, which affects health professionals as much as it affects patients.

The most significant contribution doctors make to the economy is keeping people like Suzy and Pauline out of hospital. In practice they often serve as employed technicians rather than entrepreneurs who can provide insight into how healthcare can be most effective. In many cases, only 20% of patients benefit from research because of the risk of failure in the seven steps before that research is reflected in practice.

The decisions made in the consult can be influenced by how the doctor feels, what the doctor believes and what the doctor hears (or fails to hear). How a doctor performs in practice is rarely considered a reflection of what they learn from their immediate peers and their lived personal experience.

Doctors are often required to serve in ways that are less about treating disease and more about serving society's need for custodians of scarce resources. In recent years and to some extent in response to pressure from doctors in some countries, some of these roles have changed. But those changes have diminished the connection between doctors and their patients. Doctors have been challenged consistently throughout the decades, with bureaucracy, fear of complaints and workloads featuring at the top of the list.

Behind closed doors, doctors still get to practice the art of doctoring in ways that affect the results they achieve. It's these choices that are immediately amenable to change, despite the other challenges they face.

After leaving high school, it takes seven or eight years for someone to become a qualified doctor. Their record as an undergraduate student in a preliminary science or arts degree is considered, as is their performance in the medical school entry exam.

By the time they apply to medical school their portfolio includes an impressive array of extracurricular activities. Stellar sporting or arts achievements may well help them secure that coveted place in medical school. The process is competitive, and the demand is high, with hundreds (and sometimes thousands) of people applying for a few available spots.

Yet there's growing concern about the lack of resilience among medical students accustomed to receiving guaranteed rewards for hard work. As Dr Peter Gray was told by the head of counselling services at a major university:

> *"Students are afraid to fail; they do not take risks;*
> *they need to be certain about things. For many of*
> *them, failure is seen as catastrophic and unacceptable.*
> *External measures of success are more important than*
> *learning and autonomous development."[103]*

Qualifying as a doctor begins another long spell of training and examination. Postgraduate students face the added challenge of working long hours as a junior doctor while studying for yet more exams. To get into the specialty of their choice, doctors spend years:

- competing with their peers
- sustaining demanding jobs
- raising families
- negotiating exams few manage to pass on their first attempt

There are more doctors in the world now than at any time in the past.[104] Yet in many countries new doctors—apparently the brightest, most resourceful and most creative young people—are unemployed or struggling to find jobs.[105] Those who *do* find work may find it challenging to get beyond first base to their preferred specialist training position.

The best and brightest doctors work hard in a competitive environment with no certainty their efforts will be rewarded—financially or otherwise. They must also contend with cost-cutting measures throughout their careers because the paymaster is always concerned about the runaway cost of medicine.

We're training more doctors than ever before but it has created an oversupply of doctors in some geographical areas and a shortage in other areas where life and work can be more challenging. Specialties such as general practice (family medicine) that are vital to the future of healthcare are less attractive than high-tech specialties, particularly those based in university teaching hospitals in central business districts or urban centres of larger cities.[106] As a result, we have doctors who don't have the necessary preparation to attend to people like Suzy, Joe and Fran who are found in many (if not most) specialities.

People whose problems defy an easy fix or need help have to contend with a healthcare system that's struggling to serve them.

Some junior doctors enter their careers expecting their coveted medical degree to retain its value in income and prestige. However, after completing their training they soon learn a medical degree inducts them mainly into the service of those most vulnerable—the dependent and the dying. Rather than the smiling, happy people depicted in the hospital's brochures, these people are more likely to be distressed and unhappy.

The rewards in medicine don't always reflect how 'special' doctors are in any tangible way. There are no awards for caring in a society where the consumer is king. Doctors often have to bear the displeasure of people like Frank and Jonathan who resent the rules that limit their access to drugs and tests. They must also attend to patients who believe they know what they need or are accustomed to getting what they want.

Doctors who don't have the resilience to deal with negative feedback or can't cope with failing to 'cure' every patient face a lifetime of challenges. Such a perspective can corrode their commitment to years of selfless service.

Many find the reality of their chosen career a lot different to what they imagined and will result in one of three outcomes:

- rediscovering the art of medicine
- burning out
- leaving the profession

In the meantime, doctors may find themselves living and working in communities that expect them to live in upmarket homes, drive new cars, take foreign holidays and send their children to private schools. These luxuries come at a cost and the resulting debts can force them into a lifetime of servitude.

## *Scarcity and doctors*

It can be frustrating when the solution to a patient's problem is 'obvious,' but the patient can't seem to make the 'right' choice. This frustration is most prevalent in 'deprived' communities where doctors need to be the most proactive and patients seem the least likely to take their 'professional' advice.[107] This can result in a steady stream of healthcare professionals moving on, having experienced 'scarcity' in serving people with complex and seemingly intractable social problems.

These three scarcities (time, resources and resilience) create what Julian Tudor Hart calls the inverse care law.[108]

> *A higher propensity of GP burnout was found among GPs with a high share of deprived patients on their lists compared to GPs with a low share of deprived patients. This applied in particular to patients on social benefits. This indicates that besides lower supply of GPs in deprived areas, people in these areas may also be served by GPs who are in higher risk of burnout and not performing optimally.[109]*

Loosely summarised, the inverse care law states that services are provided the least where they're needed the most. In areas where I encountered a large proportion of patients like Suzy, Mildred, Hamish or Fran, the clinics would lose doctors after a few years (and sometimes a few months).

Doctors who most need to serve patients in creative ways to improve their outcomes might consider framing their patients' needs in the context of scarcity.[110] It's almost impossible to 'motivate' Suzy to make different choices when she has competing demands for her limited financial and psychological resources.

We need to revisit the healthcare paradigm and treat those who seem to be making poor choices as victims of scarcity rather than being unintelligent or unwilling. In doing so we may need to 'vaccinate' healthcare professionals against the dangers of this environment eroding their skills and commitment. We may not be able to change the circumstances in which patients such as Suzy and Joanna turn to doctors for help. But we can start recognising how those doctors respond to their needs.

If medicine is a partnership between doctor and patient, then so are the results. As always, context is everything and the way the doctor presents in that encounter is a crucial component.

The late American paediatrician Barbara Starfield's ideas still resonate with many who work in primary care. Family doctors serve to reduce costs in a healthcare system by keeping people like Joe out of hospital.[111]

Having said that, the probability of your family doctor needing to make a heroic effort such as saving Ryan from being poisoned is very low, as patients are more likely to be suffering from a cold than a more serious infection or a poisoning.

The best a doctor can do is reassure the patient that the pain, rash, cough, discharge or fever will resolve itself in a few days.[112] They may recommend an over-the-counter painkiller, rest or exercise. Above all they will tell the patient to be… well, patient.

As a patient you'll either leave the room feeling better or get a second opinion at the hospital emergency department. Either way, it will influence how you feel about going back to that doctor and whether it was worth the dollars you/the insurance company/the government invested in that visit.

## *When things go wrong*

To the casual observer, it can seem 'obvious' why things go wrong in medicine. For example, why are only a few people with a heart defect prescribed a life-saving drug? Everyone has an opinion:

- "Doctors don't follow the recommended guidelines."
- "Patients don't take their medicine."
- "People can't afford such expensive drugs."
- "Doctors aren't doing their jobs properly."

And the truth may encompass any, all or none of them.

Let's do some math, using the evidence-to-practice pipeline developed by Glasziou and Haynes, for these seven steps:[113]

1. Doctors are aware of the research or guidelines.
2. Doctors accept the evidence underpinning these guidelines.
3. Doctors remember to apply the guidelines when the relevant patients seek their help.
4. It is possible to do something practical to comply with the guidelines.
5. Doctors act to offer the relevant treatment.

6. Doctors and patients agree on the need for that treatment.

7. Patients comply with the treatment.

If we assume 80% adherence for each step, then only 21% ($0.8 \times 0.8 \times 0.8 \times 0.8 \times 0.8 \times 0.8 \times 0.8 = 0.21$) of people with the relevant problem will be managed according to 'the guidelines.' Experience also suggests that in many if not most conditions, only one in five people will be managed as per expert recommendations.

A quick review of the literature more or less confirms this prediction:

- Only 17% of patients with diabetes were screened for sexual dysfunction despite it being a common complication of this condition.[114]

- The proportion of treated patients whose blood pressure was controlled to < 160/90 mm Hg remained at only 33%.[115]

- When examining the referral origin of all colorectal cancer patients, only 24% were referred 'urgently' according to national guidelines.[116]

An agile and cost-effective solution could be devised for any problem in medicine providing we consider how it's deployed. Doctors already have some of the necessary credentials—they're present in every encounter with a patient and they often conduct dozens of consultations every day. We could also devise a solution using creativity and logic that changes the way everyone involved feels when they're doing what's necessary.

So, how do doctors make decisions?

## *What helps doctors decide?*

Family doctors are the most often consulted health service providers in Australia and many other countries. In 2010–11, an estimated 14.5 million Australians aged 15 years and over (82% of the population) visited such a doctor at least once in the previous year, with 11.8 million having more than one consultation.[117] At the time, the 43,400 family doctors (aka general practitioners or GPs) in Australia worked an average of 42 hours per week. A 2015 census reported that the average age of a GP was 49.3, with almost one in three older than 55.[118] Yet studies seldom report the effect a doctor's age has on the advice they offer in their practice.

If tailoring healthcare advice to the patient's ideas and expectations is important then we also need to consider the personal experiences of the healthcare professional providing the service. For example, we know whether Joe receives evidence-based care will be influenced less by lectures, guidelines and protocols targeting doctors and more by:

- clinic staffroom conversations
- peer pressure
- the views of opinion leaders
- personal experience within a doctor's circle of influence[119]

In research on innovations delivered in the consultation, the clinician is a significant confounding variable and a limitation researchers rarely acknowledge.

> *"Primary care clinicians work in 'communities of practice,' combining information from a wide range of sources into 'mindlines' (internalised, collectively reinforced tacit guidelines), which they use to inform their practice."[120]*

As an example, a recent report demonstrated that the diagnosis and treatment of malaria was significantly impacted by what doctors thought appropriate notwithstanding what was urged by the guidelines.

> *"Despite recent efforts that have been made to improve access to diagnostic tools and to reduce the overuse of antimalarials, there is still considerable antimalarial drugs pressure at the population level. Improving rational use of drugs is necessary to prevent the development of resistance. The present findings indicate that the goal of the WHO guidelines of systematic diagnostic testing and treatment upon result is far from being reached and that antimalarial treatments are not targeted to the individuals in need."[123]*

Also, doctors don't necessarily follow clinical guidelines when treating themselves or their families.[121]

So, what would make doctors more likely to provide evidence-based care for chronic and complex conditions? With one in three GPs over 55, many of them will be experiencing the onset of chronic illness—diabetes, lower back pain, depression, cancer, etc.—along with their partners, families and friends. They'll also be likely targets for screening tests, particularly colorectal and breast cancer, in many countries.

A doctor's attitudes and experiences may well predict how they treat their patients. For example, when Anders Beach and colleagues asked doctors for their views on screening patients for alcohol abuse, they didn't ask participating doctors about their own experiences with alcohol, or the experiences of close family or friends. One participating practitioner said, "To me, just asking everybody about their drinking habits is in part comparable to if I had to do a rectal examination on all patients that came to see me."[122]

Everyone assumes doctors will always provide evidence-based advice. In reality, as BJ Fogg's behaviour theory suggests, the outcome of a consultation depends on the alignment of three factors: motivation, ability and trigger.[123] Assuming the most appropriate treatment is available and the doctor is allowed to offer it, what factors will affect their motivation to provide this advice?

## *Time*

The time patients spend with their GPs during initial consultations is declining. According to a study published in the Australian Healthcare and Hospitals Association's journal:

> *The proportion of GPs providing 'Level C'*
> *consultations (longer than 20 minutes) is substantial*
> *(96%) and constant; however, the number of lengthy*
> *consultations provided per GP decreased by 21%*
> *between 2006 and 2010. The proportion of GPs*
> *providing Level D consultations (longer than 40*

> *minutes) decreased from 72% in 2006 to 62% in*
> *2009, while the number of Level D consultations*
> *provided per GP decreased by 26%.[124]*

Meanwhile, the number of problems presented to doctors is increasing. In a survey of 8,707 patients sampled from 290 GPs, approximately half of them had two or more chronic conditions.[125]

The time available for routine doctor-patient meetings is often limited not only by the number of problems patients present, but also by the need to:

- record the consultation for legal and administrative reasons
- collect data electronically

Doctors can spend more time entering information on a screen than looking at patients like Joe, Suzy, Joanna and Pauline because they'll all present a multitude of issues that need to be documented.

As much as technology has improved healthcare, it has also reduced the scope to offer such patients undivided attention. Doctors are also less likely to physically examine Jonathan because the tests and scans are readily available. The value of the examination in not only gathering clinical information but also nourishing an emotional connection between doctor and patient is being undermined.[126]

The very foundations of doctoring are being eroded to increase administrative efficiency, or to vainly find the needle of pathology (as for Fran) in the haystack of consultations.

In the commercially driven world of convenience and speed, the internet now provides easy access to doctors or health practitioners with a ready prescription pad or test request. A host of service providers promoted by commercial interests now use the internet to provide access to advice, prescriptions and referrals. Telehealth now affects every country in the West and is increasingly affecting developing countries as well. It's been called the 'ATM' of the medical world, with the scope to revolutionise the healthcare industry.

Curiously, many people now look for alternative and complementary health services that offer more face-to-face time and focus more on the experience than conventional healthcare, which seems to be more and more about exchanging money for a prescription, referral or test.

## *Muffin Power*

It was 2014 and I was standing in the waiting room at what was purportedly one of the best teaching practices in a major city.

But according to the receptionist, we weren't fully prepared for the visit.

"If you haven't brought morning tea [a midmorning snack] then they [the doctors] won't see you," she said.

I was speechless and the researchers accompanying me were mortified.

"But I'm not a pharmaceutical company representative. I'm a fellow general practitioner and a professor at a local university, invited here by one of your doctors to discuss a research project. My team and I have travelled an hour across the city to get here."

"I'm sorry," she insisted, "but the doctors expect morning tea before they see any representatives."

With time running out for my appointment I dashed out, vaulted over a fence to a nearby petrol station, and bought a dozen muffins. The sugary baked goods were duly taken to the tearoom while I waited on the other side of the reception desk.

The doctors filed in to examine my offering. Clearly, they didn't pass muster, as only one of the five doctors I came to see stayed to speak with me. The rest decided they were 'too busy', although they stood in the corridor for a long time before filing away to their rooms to do whatever they were too busy doing to spend 10 minutes hearing why I'd been invited by one of their peers.

I wondered how well paid, caring and successful people now needed to be bribed with sweet treats. If pharmaceutical company representatives made a habit of offering bribes, how did it affect the doctors' prescribing habits?

The evidence presented by Moynihan, Heath, and Henry (2002) is disconcerting.

> *Disease mongering can include turning ordinary*
> *ailments into medical problems, seeing mild symptoms*
> *as serious, treating personal problems as medical,*
> *seeing risks as diseases, and framing prevalence*
> *estimates to maximise potential markets.*[127]

It's been suggested that potentially dangerous drugs are promoted by an industry whose leaders reportedly dream of their products becoming as widely used as chewing gum.[128] With healthcare policy encouraging doctors to see as many patients as possible, some doctors are seduced into deploying their prescription pads to get through the day. The pharmaceutical industry has achieved this by deploying the same tactics used to get any 'consumer' to buy—not as a purchaser, but as an agent.

> *With rare exceptions, studies of exposure to information provided directly by pharmaceutical companies have found associations with higher prescribing frequency, higher costs, or lower prescribing quality or have not found significant associations. We did not find evidence of net improvements in prescribing, but the available literature does not exclude the possibility that prescribing may sometimes be improved.[129]*

Factors that affect decisions made during a visit to a doctor can be summarised under three headings:

- How the doctor feels
- What the doctor believes
- What the doctor hears (or fails to hear)

These factors are typically hard to influence, so ideas that will have the greatest effect rarely focus on increasing motivation to provide specific treatments. Therefore, innovations aimed at changing what doctors do seldom work.

The literature identifies several specific factors:

## Complaints

*An overwhelming majority of respondents (91.0%)
reported believing that physicians order more tests
and procedures than needed to protect themselves from
malpractice suits. These views were consistent across a
range of physician characteristics, most notably across
specialty groups, where 91.2% of generalists, 88.6%
of medical specialists, 92.5% of surgeons, and 93.8%
of other specialists agreed with the statement
(P = .35). No significant differences were seen by
geographic location, type of practice, or professional
society affiliation.*[130]

## The doctor's experience or training

* *Widely used Continuing Medical Education (CME)
delivery methods such as conferences have little direct
impact on improving professional practice. More
effective methods such as systematic practice-based
interventions and outreach visits are seldom used by
CME providers.*[131]

It's been shown that doctors don't necessarily keep up with
the latest research. Their knowledge in particular may erode
over time. That means that within a few years of completing
their training, doctors may already be out of step with what's
known about their topic.[132]

On closer inspection, they may continue with practices
closer to the custom and practice of when they completed
their training. This might seem catastrophic, except most

people who visit a family doctor are most likely to have a self-limiting condition or are simply worried. Others, such as Suzy and Joanna, rarely act on advice.

Other factors that affect doctors' opinions are:

## Perceptions

*A total of 4845 discrete items were mentioned as being capable of influencing Family Physicians' (FPs') decisions about referral for consultation. Aggregation of related items resulted in a list of 35 nonmedical factors, of which 11 were identified by at least half the respondents and 14 by less than half but more than 10. These 25 factors fell into three categories: patient and family factors (e.g., patient's wishes), FP and consultant factors (e.g., FP's capabilities), and other influences (e.g., style of practice). On the basis of both the frequency of identification and priority scores "patient's wishes" emerged as the most important factor.[133]*

## Payment structures

*The use of financial incentives to reward Primary Care Practitioners for improving the quality of primary healthcare services is growing. However, there is insufficient evidence to support or not support the use of financial incentives to improve the quality of primary health care.[134]*

## The doctor's mood

*82 doctors reported recent incidents where they considered that symptoms of stress had negatively affected their patient care. The qualitative accounts they gave were coded for the attribution (type of stress symptom) made, and the effect it had. Half of these effects concerned lowered standards of care; 40% were the expression of irritability or anger; 7% were serious mistakes which still avoided directly leading to death, and two resulted in patient death. The attributions given for these were largely to do with tiredness (57%) and the pressure of overwork (28%), followed by depression or anxiety (8%), and the effects of alcohol (5%).[135]*

## Time of day

*The researchers looked at the billing and electronic health record (EHR) data for patient visits to 23 different primary care practices over the course of 17 months. Then identified visit diagnoses using billing codes and, using EHRs, identified visit times, antibiotic prescriptions and chronic illnesses. They analysed over 21-thousand Acute Respiratory Infections visits by adults, which occurred during two four-hour sessions, 8 a.m. to noon and 1 p.m. to 5 p.m. The researchers found that antibiotic prescribing increased throughout the morning and afternoon clinic sessions.[136]*

## Multiple problems

*In many healthcare systems, providers see patients during brief office visits and are overwhelmed by the number of health maintenance activities recommended by guidelines and quality monitoring agencies. When diabetic patients have multiple chronic conditions, screening, counselling, and treatment needs far exceed the time available for patient–provider visits.*[137]

## Cultural differences

*Most clinicians lack the information to understand how culture influences the clinical encounter and the skills to bridge potential differences effectively. New strategies are required to expand medical training to adequately address culturally discordant encounters among the physicians, their patients, and the families, for all three may have different concepts regarding the nature of the disease, expectations about treatment, and modes of appropriate communication beyond language.*[138]

## Distractions in the consultation

*The presence of the computer has changed the beginning of the consultation. Where once only two actors needed to perform their roles, now three interact in differing ways. Information comes from many sources, and behaviour responds accordingly. Future studies of the consultation need to take into*

*account the impact of the computer in shaping how the*
*consultation flows and the information needs of*
*all participants.*[139]

## Other roles

Certain duties that were once a significant part of the doctor's role have changed beyond recognition over the past couple of decades. In the past, particularly in the UK, doctors also consulted with patients in their homes, both during and after office hours.[140] The right to be seen at home if you weren't 'fit to travel' was enshrined in payment structures. Any patient with a bad cold could make a case for not travelling on the basis that it could be something more serious and pose a risk to their wellbeing or the welfare of others.

In some instances, the home's condition significantly limited the scope for examinations, particularly physical examinations. Angela's home was a difficult place to properly examine a feverish child and a dimly lit hallway is a challenging place to determine the cause of a sore throat in a seemingly healthy teenager like Ryan.

At the time, people believed their doctor would take care of them from birth to death—24 hours a day, 365 days a year. Some members of the profession were against jettisoning the need for doctors to do home visits, especially visits outside office hours. They insisted that home visits were a fundamental cornerstone of doctoring and the profession could claim to be unique among health service providers in their understanding of patients.[141]

The requirement to do home visits came at a great cost to doctors, who were already contending with:

- the stress of increased workloads
- busy roads
- a lack of parking in sprawling urban centres
- patients like Angela who were getting used to whatever convenience was on offer

With the rising incidence of substance abuse, a number of doctors were also physically attacked by people under the influence of drugs. A few were even murdered while visiting patients.

The risks and inefficiency appeared to outweigh the benefits.

The doctors' service contract with the funder was revised with great fanfare. It was no longer necessary for doctors to be 'on call' to patients. It also decoupled a primary emotional link between doctors and patients. The home of general practice—the heartland of a profession that provided continuity of care where geography and timing were no barrier—was changed forever. It could be strongly argued the change was inevitable as demography, expectations and circumstances have morphed. However, the doctors' preoccupations of bureaucracy, fear of complaints and poor work-life balance have remained consistent throughout the decades.[142]

On the other hand, the literature documents the rise of so-called alternative providers, who are growing in popularity and profitability despite the lack of an evidence base.[143] Doctors have noticed that patients may be willing to pay for alternative treatments—even treatments that have no research evidence and could even harm them.[144] In this context, Jonathan could fall prey to the outrageous claims of a vitamin supplier. Even in countries where the state subsidises access to doctors, people appear reticent to fork out a few dollars to see one.

Wellbeing has now been packaged as a commodity that can be doled out at speed by anyone in a sanitised space claiming expertise, wearing a white coat and brandishing that most iconic medical instrument—the stethoscope.

As custodians of limited resources, doctors are also expected to be leaders and innovators. They receive little or no training in this regard but are still expected to get the best out of their staff and ensure their practice is effective, safe and efficient.[145]

However, in their professional role doctors are more often cast as technicians and employees rather than entrepreneurs, managers or artists—even though they're among the most creative, diligent and resourceful people I've ever met. Most had to prove as much just to get into medical school.

This creativity can be frustrated or sublimated, or it can be harnessed to re-engineer evidence-based medicine and deliver better care. In the status quo, every symptom is framed as a biomedical puzzle that can only be solved with dozens of tests. To realise the value of our investment in the healthcare sector, we need a better way to deploy the intuition, insight, empathy and creativity of healers.

The doctor is a key stakeholder in the economy of healthcare, not only as a professional but also with respect to their personal history and prejudices. Framing healthcare this way has implications for treatment as well as diagnosis.

If we accept that patients need to be seen and heard, then if the doctor's senses are jaundiced by their personal history, their assessment of needs, symptom severity and risk could be off target. If the doctors Frank and Joe consulted were overweight, they might have thought Frank and Joe's growing girths were acceptable. To help innovators, we need empirical evidence that addressing this question in a defined setting can deliver better outcomes for patients.

A healthcare organisation employs many doctors who have nothing to do with its policies but still get to choose what they wear. Chances are someone else owns the building, pays the bills, chooses the furniture and wallpaper, employs the staff, writes the policies and sets the opening hours. But during the consultation there are only two people in the room: the doctor and the patient.

The doctor gets to choose:

- their mood
- how they greet the patient
- how they introduce themselves
- where they sit in the room[146]
- where they look during the meeting
- when they stop talking or interrupting
- whether they examine the patient
- what they focus on during the meeting
- what they say and how they say it
- their response to the assessment of information at hand
- how they end the consultation

In contrast, all patients get to do most of the time is decide whether they like it.

Doctors get to choose much of what matters to a patient. And that choice can make a big difference. Patients make choices based on how they feel—choices that determine the effect their illness has on their families, their employers and the economy.

So how can we maintain and grow the link between doctors and their patients? What could regenerate the sense of them sharing a unique and powerful bond? It's unlikely that widespread home visiting will remain or be introduced in many subsidised health services. That means the office encounter needs to evolve instead. To spur on that evolution, we must review every aspect of the encounter.

# 7

# THE STAGE

The art of doctoring is performed on a stage where people interact, and decisions are made.

Most complaints about healthcare services relate to how patients are made to feel rather than their diagnosis or treatment. Also, the places where healthcare is provided have a major influence on how they feel.

Unfortunately, they've hardly changed in decades. Most clinics are similar to a government bureaucracy outpost, with décor and furniture that wouldn't look out of place in a bus terminal—hardly the place to inspire Suzy or Jonathan to make better choices.

In surveys about subsidised services, respondents said they wouldn't be willing to pay very much to visit their family doctor. And yet 'alternative and complementary health practitioners' with little evidence base to back them up are flourishing.

In this chapter I'll use the 'Value Tunnel' as a framework to explain why conventional health services have a lower perceived value than other flourishing commercial experiences.

The demographic groups that visit doctors most often are women, older people and parents with young children. Their experience from the moment they enter the building is often unfriendly, forbidding and impersonal. By framing their experience as a commercial business, healthcare providers can think of every interaction with them as an opportunity to add value. No connection means no added value and no sale.

Front of house staff (receptionists and medical assistants) must understand the enormous difference they make in the experience of visiting the doctor. These staff often hear the patient's reason for their visit, as well as their impression of that visit.

This information is gold.

As well as providing vital information about patient perceptions, they also have the opportunity to promote health and wellbeing. The business of healthcare appears to be based on efficiently making claims for services rendered on behalf of insurers or for government subsidies. There's little incentive to provide anything more than a room or virtual space for people to receive the consultations three main outputs: tests, prescriptions and referrals. Framing the art of doctoring as the business of doctoring makes healthcare ripe for disruption.

In many countries, the way family doctors are set up to serve patients has hardly changed since the first clinic opened more than a century ago. This issue received recent attention in medical literature, with authors concluding that "96 percent of patient complaints are related to customer service, while only 4 percent are about the quality of clinical care or misdiagnoses."[147]

This chapter relates to the premises where doctors see their patients—not just the building, but also how people are processed through it.

Except in dire emergencies, people make appointments and sit in waiting rooms to spend a few minutes with a clinician in an office-style environment. While medical technology had advanced in leaps and bounds, the business practices and customer service of doctors has barely evolved. New practices still look like bus stations divided into small partitioned rooms. They create an atmosphere similar to a government department, which is unlikely to make patients 'feel' better.

When asked how much they're willing to pay for a visit to a doctor (particularly a generalist), most people place little value on the experience.

> *One hundred forty-seven college students and 58 senior citizens viewed 35 slides of physicians' waiting rooms. Using a visual analog scale, participants rated the perceived quality of care and the environment of each waiting room. The primary hypothesis was that perceived quality of care would be greater for waiting rooms that were nicely furnished, well-lighted, contained artwork, and warmer in appearance versus waiting rooms that had outdated furnishings, were dark, contained no artwork or poor-quality reproductions, and were cold in appearance. Factor analyses of the care and environment ratings produced factors consistent with the hypothesis.[148]*

Australians spend more than $4 billion each year on complementary and alternative medicine (CAM) and visit CAM practitioners almost as frequently as they do medical practitioners. And the spending doesn't stop there.

> *The national survey of Australians (18–64 years) found over the past four weeks Australians spent an average of $594 each on clothes, accessories, beauty products and cosmetic services. Victoria, the self-proclaimed fashion capital of Australia, is home to the biggest spenders, who spend 19 per cent more than the national average at $707 a month. New South Wales spent $669 on average, 13 per cent more than average, followed by South Australia ($618) and Western Australia ($616).[149]*

Comparatively, a family doctor or GP might charge $50 for a standard consultation. The Medicare rebate (the Australian government subsidy for a consultation with a family doctor) is $36.30, leaving a gap of $13.70 for the patient to pay out of their own pockets—about the cost of a café breakfast at an average Melbourne restaurant. Across Australia, the average out-of-pocket amount for an adult visiting a GP is $29.56 a year.

In Australia, New Zealand and the UK, patients will usually see their doctor in a converted residential or commercial space that was once a shop, someone's home or a repurposed office. There will mostly like be a reception area and waiting room, with the receptionist (usually female) sitting behind a tall counter or glass window.

The waiting room will have plastic bucket seats along the walls, a few coffee tables with old magazines stacked on them and perhaps a box of donated toys in the corner. There may also be a television on a wall either playing 'information videos' or screening daytime television.

The floors covering will be commercial carpet, tiles or lino. The room will have posters describing various symptoms, treatments and health advice either stuck to the walls or pinned to a board. There will be leaflets on everything from child immunisation and blood pressure checks to cancer screening tests and the signs of a stroke will be on offer.

In other words, it will have the look and feel of somewhere you'd go to renew a driving license or lodge a tax return and all the atmosphere of an airport gate lounge.

There will be no obvious smell, but plenty of sound— patients making appointments or negotiating with staff and telephones ringing constantly, almost demanding to be answered. The receptionist or medical assistant will juggle various demands while churning through masses of paperwork to process the day's influx of patients. When the phone rings, they'll typically state the name of the clinic and then ask the caller to hold. Behind them, in an area lit by the glow of their computer screens, printers will spit out reams of paper.

Those waiting will glance at their mobile devices or make calls despite the signs urging people to switch them off. Those who *do* switch them off (or don't have one) will stare at the television, leaf through a book or magazine or check their watches.

Children will play on the floor or pester a harried parent whenever their name isn't called. And everyone will avoid contact until their names are called and they're led to a doctor's office.

In many countries, the doctor's room will look like any office apart from perhaps a couch and a trolley with a few instruments. But in the UK and Australia the doctor will probably be sitting seated in a high-back chair behind a desk cluttered with paperwork, pharmaceutical company leaflets, cheap pens, faxes and notices from the health department and a computer and printer nestled beside the phone.

In other countries the patient may be propped up on an examination couch, with the doctor either sitting on a stool with castors or standing by the bed. Family members accompanying the patient will be asked to sit beside the patient or in a corner of the room, often in noticeably smaller seats.

The patient might hear a sick child complaining, a printer at work or people walking along the corridor to other rooms. There may be a smell of disinfectant or air freshener, or the musty whiff of old office furniture.

The cluttered pile of equipment on display may include:

- a stethoscope
- an auroscope
- a tendon hammer
- an electronic sphygmomanometer
- a box of sterile gloves

There may also be a trolley loaded with clinic room equipment in sealed plastic bags, the drawers stocked with specimen bottles, needles, syringes and other paraphernalia.

If you're booked for a procedure or vaccination in the UK or Australia, you may be ushered into a nurse's treatment room with a large adjustable clinic room bed (similar to a hospital treatment room). It will also have a kitchen style counter with neatly stacked boxes full of dressings and other bits and pieces.

The room may have a couch (examination table) with a light mounted above it and a small desk and chair in the corner with a computer on the desk (unless the health professional prefers glancing at an iPad).

You may also see a defibrillator screwed onto the wall and a luridly coloured plastic box covered in warnings for the safe disposal of used needles.

(In the US, this room is probably where you'd see the doctor.)

This style of 'clinic' or variations on the theme can be found in suburban centres in the towns, cities and villages of many developed countries. Depending on where you live, there could be several of them on the one block.

While there's no reliable count, there are thought to be around 4,000 such clinics in Australia. In the UK, they'd be part of the doctor's home that was converted so they could see their queue of patients in a businesslike way.

In the 1950s there were movements to set up community health centres modelled on hospital clinics, which were set up similarly so patients could efficiently attend them for technical fixups. They were places patients could go for prescriptions, injections, tests and referrals without having to discuss their health more broadly.

There are exceptions to this rule. Some clinics are located in architecturally designed, light-filled, award-winning premises with widescreen televisions, filtered water, thick pile carpets and piped-in music. But they follow the same principles of every other clinic: the patient makes an appointment to meet a doctor for a brief consultation and at the end they receive a prescription, certificate or test order.

The model that's barely changed in a century and is designed to be as efficient as possible rather than to enhance the experience of the user.

While people might be willing to spend $100 for a massage or $90 for a haircut, they'll baulk at paying even a third of that amount to see a family doctor or GP. In most countries, specialists are even more expensive because you can't access them directly.

As an alternative to visiting their local doctor, some people may choose to:

- pick one that doesn't charge more than the government rebate
- visit a pharmacy
- go to an emergency department

Hairdressers can charge as much as they do because there are limited alternatives to getting a haircut from 'that' salon or 'that' hairdresser. But there's constant downward pressure in this tunnel and as competition in the market increases, the prices fall. That's why a coffee costs about $5 and isn't perceived as being worth any more than that.

So, what can GPs do to increase their perceived value? What could help them earn more in a niche market? While doctors no longer hold the monopoly on a lot of things, they can still offer services that others can't provide. How can family doctors recast their brand in a way that will sustain (if not enhance) their perceived value to patients?

Like every other business, healthcare is subject to market forces. A recent survey offered businesses the following takeaways to handle those market forces:[150]

- **Know your customer and form a genuine relationship.** What do the doctors or other staff know about their patients that isn't limited to routinely collected data on bodily function? How is that information used? Given that the clinic collects the patient's birthdate. How is that information used to identify teachable moments?

- **Make it easy for your customers to do business with you.** To what extent can patients access what they need at the clinic? For example, what happens when there's an emergency at the clinic and the doctor is running behind schedule?

- **Solve your customer's problems and go beyond what is expected.** To what extent is the clinic a one-stop shop? What does the practice offer that other providers don't? (Note: pharmacists and online consultations don't offer physical examinations.)

- **Look for opportunities to make an impression.** Does the practice communicate well with patients at every touchpoint?
- **Invest in your frontline staff; they are of course the face of your company, so it is essential that they happily reflect the core values you wish to promote.** What are the reception staff and medical assistants like? Can patients expect to be treated with respect by everyone they come across at the clinic?

Patients will use doctors to a different extent at different points in their lives. Most children will see a doctor several times in their early years—usually for immunisation, but also when they succumb to one of the many minor infections common in early childhood.

In later childhood and early adulthood people are less likely to attend doctors' clinics, the one exception being women of childbearing age who present for contraceptive advice or antenatal care.

The consultation rates pick up again in middle and late middle age, as patients such as Pauline and Frank develop long-term and life-limiting illnesses.

The heaviest users of healthcare are older people with established conditions, who may attend as often as twice a month.

Consultation rates also vary depending on where the practice is located.[151] In 'deprived' communities they may be higher than in more affluent areas, although in those communities the rates may also be lower due to a relative shortage of doctors.

One would also expect the outcomes to be worse in some areas. This may be true for life-limiting illness, but there's evidence to suggest outcomes may also be poor in areas that are relatively well served with doctors.[152] The differences in outcomes may reflect the way care is provided as well as the quality of that care.

## The experience

While most people will visit their local clinic, and usually during office hours, the 'parking' facilities may still be unsatisfactory.[153] For patients who *do* get parked, their first point of contact when entering the premises is usually some sort of a barrier such as a tall desk or glass window, which sends the wrong message:

- You're on that side and we are on this side.
- We're hiding things from you back here.
- You're here to 'get something' from us, but we're not sure we want you here just now.
- We're very busy and your needs are one of the many things we have to cope with today.

Designing the 'ideal' reception counter involves a number of steps. But the first step should be considering what is needed in the first place.

> *What kind of impression should it make? Should it be warm and inviting, or bold and austere? What kind of reaction do you want to create in the visitor? Is it purely functional or a real 'statement piece' aimed at dominating the whole area?[154]*

The counters in many practices seem to be designed to process a queue, much like the counter at an airport check-in or a vehicle licensing office. It speaks to why the clinic thinks it's necessary to have it.

> *Who will be using it from the visitor side? Will it be treated with respect by all who come into contact with it, or must it be able to withstand some abuse? Maybe a tough, metallic finish would help to prolong the counter's working life.*[155]

When a patient arrives, they must:

1. check in
2. prove they're entitled to be there (i.e. that they have an appointment)
3. prove they can pay or are insured, or make a payment right away
4. state their business succinctly and clearly

The counter conceals computer terminals, printers, fax machines and security equipment. It's also there to protect staff and preserve privacy. To complete the 'look,' the walls may be covered in mismatching posters and the counter stocked with a leaflet dispenser filled to the brim.

However, there's limited evidence these accessories have any useful impact.[156] In fact, evidence from the retail industry suggests that less is more.

As for the counter, it's generally as tall as it can be.

> *An able-bodied visitor with a typical minimum*
> *height of 1540mm approaching a raised counter tall*
> *enough to hide a large monitor on a desktop height*
> *of 740mm, would undoubtedly struggle to make eye*
> *contact with a seated receptionist. As a rough guide, a*
> *counter height of over 1200mm will create a potential*
> *'blind spot' resulting in the visitor remaining almost*
> *unseen and making the counter simply too high to be*
> *practical for signing in.[157]*

But what if the reception counter was removed altogether? It's not unthinkable if hotel chains are considering it.

> *Two bloggers walk into a hotel ...No, that's not*
> *the opening line to a joke. We're talking about two*
> *travellers who picked the same hotel chain—Andaz, a*
> *boutique Hyatt property. One stayed at a Los Angeles*
> *Andaz, the other at a New York City Andaz. Neither*
> *lobby contained a front desk—a growing hospitality-*
> *industry trend that's equal parts chic and shrewd.[158]*

There are umpteen reasons why clinic reception counters are traditionally designed as described, the main one being to simplify payment processing. Other industries that perform similar administrative tasks are striving for better solutions rather than barricading patients and sending the wrong message.

Here's an insightful comment from a 'front of house' staff member:

*Our role has developed from "just scheduling staff" to
a more complex, and crucial, role for any healthcare
organisation. We are the start and end of every patient
visit and also the start of the revenue cycle. In order
for "customer service" to improve, an organisation
must first recognise the importance of their Patient
Access department and understand that their processes
are directly related to the culture of the organisation.[159]*

Is it possible that patients who feel welcome will be more
receptive to the professional advice on offer? Isn't that what
healthcare is all about? We've known this for decades. This
published quote says it all:

*The feeling in the practice when you arrive, busy...
exhausted receptionists, people fed up, waiting, a
feeling of dilapidation and stress...You can hear
people being put off on the phone and you can hear
'no no I can't put you through to the doctor now,'
'no no you'll have to call back' and that makes you
feel worse because you don't want to call back at an
inappropriate time.[160]*

The reception area creates circumstances where care
outcomes are compromised. But there's a better way and at
least one Australian practice has redesigned the experience.[161]
It has removed the reception desk and introduced desk-
mounted iPads that allow patients to check in or make
an appointment without having to bother the harassed
'multitasking' receptionist.

Patients will spend more time in the waiting room than anywhere else during their doctor visits. Waiting times for a 10-minute appointment can be 40 minutes or more at some clinics. So, they spend more time interacting with the receptionist than they do with their health practitioner. The receptionist will:

- book their appointment
- greet them on arrival
- take their details
- offer them a seat
- let the medical team know if they need to be seen to ASAP
- check them out at departure

And yet the word receptionists utter the most is "Sorry."
"Sorry about the wait."
"Sorry, we have no appointments available."
"Sorry, the doctor's running late."
Receptionists and medical assistants are well-placed to let the team know when they're failing their mission. But more importantly, they can:

- express empathy
- notice emergencies
- reduce risk (e.g. stop a child with chicken pox running around a waiting room full of soon-to-be mums)
- explain when expectations aren't being met
- defuse complaints

- maintain a sense of calm and good humour when the practice is hectic
- embody discretion and confidentiality

From the moment the patient comes into contact with the practice, receptionists can underline self-care messages and endorse what the medical team has to offer. Or they can severely compromise (if not destroy) any chance of achieving this.

Receptionists in many countries tend to be local residents (usually women), and often have little or no formal training in customer service. They're frequently left to triage calls, deciding when a call is urgent enough to interrupt the doctor or determining when someone can be slotted into a busy schedule. Also they will be the first to know whether a patient is satisfied or unhappy.

They may have been recruited after only a brief interview by the practice manager. They'll have the fewest formal qualifications of anyone in the building and be the lowest paid.[162] Yet they'll be privy to much of what the health professional will be told even before the patient enters the consulting room.

They will set the tone for each patient's experience and they're well placed to trigger health behaviours in much the same way front of house staff can influence a customer's experience in any other business.

The business of healthcare is based on efficiently generating claims for insurers or for government subsidies. There's little or no incentive to provide anything more than a place where patients can access prescriptions or tests.

Some practices will offer minor operation services to remove skin lesions or implant contraceptive devices. Most funders will offer some sort of incentive to address chronic disease management, cancer screening and other health promotion activities.

These payments made little difference in the way practices are organised overall, other than the traditional model described earlier. Patients will hear, see, smell, feel and potentially taste things that will affect whether they can disclose important information about the reason for their visit.

What patients hear is crucial, because it influences the way they'll disclose what's bothering them. The diagnosis, which underpins the treatment, is based on this information. It's important to consider what they hear during their doctor's visit.

# 8

# THE SCRIPT

The art of doctoring includes what the actors say in the Theatre Model©. The relationship between consumers and service providers is changing. With each passing generation, people are demanding more choice in decisions that affect them.

By studying human interactions, we've learnt that both what is said and the way it's said has a crucial impact on what the person with the problem will do next. What patients hear in the clinic sets the tone of their response to healthcare.

The words patients and doctors use are powerful because they have influence. The most crucial job in healthcare is to persuade people risking their future wellbeing to:

- stop smoking
- eat and drink less
- exercise more
- get screened for early detection of an increasingly long list of diseases

What a patient tells their doctor (and how they tell them) is usually the fastest way to predict the outcome of their visit. Their encounter can be heading on a particular course before the patient even enters the clinic.

It's also crucial for the advice to be delivered by the person best qualified to offer it. While there's a great deal of emphasis on verbal exchanges during the consultation, the sweetest sound is actually silence. It represents the space in which patients find the opportunity and the cue to express their ideas, concerns and expectations without judgement or interruption.

The most critical question in the theatre of the consultation is, "What's on your mind?" followed by silence.

Doctors perform best when they don't restrict the patient's disclosure or force the solution. They need to demonstrate trust and acknowledge the patients' autonomy to make choices for themselves. It may be that the context of Joe's visit hasn't been established and the doctor may not be aware he has limited health literacy or has been misguided by unreliable information online. Fran may believe her symptoms are caused by something that's scientifically impossible.

Similarly, research has shown that what Angela experiences before seeking help may dictate her responses when she meets with her doctor. This can be risky insofar as that information can be misused to promote tests or treatments driven by commercial interests.

Nonetheless, we must carefully consider when and how questions are framed, especially when offering choices to patients who are vulnerable to adverse outcomes and believe they have no choice but to accept what's on offer. Information that includes references to sex, novelty or threats can also capture their attention.

Presenting information as numerical data may be ineffective, as the patient may find numbers difficult to understand. The primary function of language isn't just to express or describe but also to persuade, which it does by signposting people to mental associations that favour the best outcome.

And that makes the script used in the theatre of the consultation vitally important in the art of doctoring.

Many years ago, I overheard a conversation in my practice that went something like this:

"Sorry Jean, but there aren't any appointments available until Friday. Has he got a fever? Try him with some paracetamol today and I'll book him in for Friday afternoon. There's a lot of this flu-like thing going around the schools. Okay, see you Friday."

The person answering the telephone was triaging my patients despite having no medical training. She looked up from the call with a pained expression. She was carrying more responsibility than her pay grade and yet this imbalance has long been recognised.

> *Little difference was observed between the symptoms reported by patients to the physicians as compared to those received by the receptionist staff. Physicians are more likely to use the telephone contact to treat the patient's complaint with home care advice or a prescription. Receptionists are more likely to use the telephone contact for scheduling an office visit.*[163]

What's rarely acknowledged is that in many settings receptionists and medical assistants (who are often recruited from the local community) take calls from friends, neighbours and relatives. The callers may be worried, unwell, confused, frustrated, angry, grieving, embarrassed, lonely, sad, suicidal, dying or simply overwhelmed.

We give these people a frontline role in a system that's often oversubscribed and understaffed. In primary care they're the first port of call for everyone who believes they need medical attention. So, it's understandable that they sometimes use words that should be reserved for healthcare professionals.[164]

We expect receptionists to be polite, courteous, discreet, sensitive, thoughtful, obliging and intuitive. But if they try to be medical and they get it wrong, the clinic could face a complaint, bad press or even litigations.

Employers have recognised the challenge inherent in the receptionist role. But in many parts of the world, those who undertake this work often have no formal qualifications or appropriate training.[165] While research has been done on this matter, there are still challenges in developing ways to help receptionist staff prioritise patients.

Can we really help someone with no medical qualifications make appropriate decisions based on a telephone conversation about potential medical emergencies? Would Ryan have had a good outcome if his sister had telephoned an inexperienced person that fateful morning? There have been examples of disastrous failures to appropriately signpost the parents of a very sick child. Some have even involved suitably qualified people working within nationally accredited algorithms.[166]

The fundamental issue is demand for access to medical practitioners outstripping supply. In response to overwhelming demand, policymakers have promoted ways to limit or control access to their expertise.

The temptation is to come up with solutions that don't require a doctor. Those who support this approach may not recognise that people in distress aren't malfunctioning machines in need of a technical fix. Their care can't be scheduled like a car service.

That doesn't mean they need to see a doctor as soon as they experience a twinge of some sort. But they need to feel they've had that experience sooner rather than later.

Patients are hardwired to feel better after contact with a doctor. It's fundamental to how medicine works.[167] When our team came to this realisation some time ago, we relieved our reception staff from having to determine who was 'not urgent for today' when our schedules were full.

Instead, our doctors spoke to those seeking urgent appointments by telephone. If we didn't think we had enough information we'd offer the patient an urgent appointment. In doing so, we reduced the demand for face-to-face appointments by 40%.

But rationing access to doctors by having someone else handle the so-called 'triage' might create more problems than it solves, if only because the patients don't think doctors care when they're worried. Patients no longer think of themselves as consumers and doctors as experts. Instead they think of themselves and the doctor as a 'team.'

People also prefer things, people, products and companies that have an association with them. This again emphasises the need to know and refer to what matters to each patient. The choices presented obviously can't take factors the patient hasn't disclosed into account and so those choices may not be in the patient's best interests. They also don't take the practitioner's own prejudices into account.

The script (i.e. what's said in the theatre of the consultation) needs to take these matters into account.

Symptoms (such as Natasha's earache) are the usual reason people consult a doctor. In fact, there's a list of symptoms most commonly presented to doctors in primary care.[168] These symptoms rarely signify a life-limiting disease, although they occasionally do as was the case with Tegan's cancer.

One of the most frequent patient complaints is not diagnosing a condition that later proves serious.[169] For this reason and because what patients tell you is often the shortest route to the correct diagnosis, the verbal exchange in the consultation is crucial. Yet doctors typically ask a closed question within seconds of the meeting.

Time pressure may drive this behaviour. The doctor may have a queue of people in the waiting room or on their appointment list for the day. So, doctors spend less time consulting with some patients—usually those with a so-called minor illness.[170] They assume the diagnosis and treatment will be straightforward, saving them time for more complex cases or perhaps to meet the demand for appointments that day.

Juliet Mavromatis offers one explanation for this pattern:

*Why do physicians interrupt? In practical terms,*
*throughout a given day a physician may be tasked*

*with listening to twenty to thirty patient-derived*
*histories and with solving difficult problems for each*
*of these patients in a matter of ten to fifteen minutes.*
*This is a tough, if not impossible job. Consequently,*
*once a physician believes that the meat of the story is*
*out there, he or she may respond and interrupt before*
*hearing details that the patient (or colleague) feels*
*are important. In more abstract terms interruption*
*is a communication strategy that reinforces physician*
*dominance in the hierarchy of the patient-physician*
*relationship.[171]*

What the patient hears in the clinic sets the tone and predicts the outcome of the consultation. While other consumer settings may have background music humming in the background, medical clinics often have other stress-inducing sounds such as ringing phones. Sometimes there's even crying and shouting. Few clinics have a soundproof waiting room. In some clinics even the doctor's offices aren't soundproof and few take steps to reduce noise.

Which means what *can* be heard may be breaching the patient's privacy.[172]

Once they're in their office, what they say and the explanations they offer are remarkably consistent. "It's a virus," may be technically correct, but that summary may not sit well with Joe who needs the doctor to validate the discomfort of a respiratory tract infection. Joe may think it's a criticism for making a fuss about a minor irritation, delivered by someone perceived as having greater status in the meeting.

The sweetest sound in the consultation is silence—the space where a patient can express their ideas, concerns and expectations without judgement or interruption. Doctors often interrupt a patient before they've even finished their first sentence at the start of the meeting.[173]

Every doctor in general practice and family medicine learns about the 'models' of the consultation. David Pendleton designed a popular model[174] that dissects the meeting into a series of communication tasks the doctor must accomplish—from establishing the reason for the visit to choosing the treatment and inviting the patient to share their other concerns.

Teresa Pawlikowska and her colleagues summarised the thinking behind such a map of the medical consultation:

> *A fundamental change in medical culture in this area has been the recognition and acceptance of the fact that the way in which health professionals communicate, on all levels, can be enhanced, irrespective of the innate and learned abilities they already possess.*[175]

Michael Bungay Stanier published a different take with his book, *The Coaching Habit: Say Less, Ask More & Change the Way You Lead Forever.*[176] In the book he says we should change the way we communicate because the main goal in healthcare is to help patients solve their own problems.

This comes at a time when the relationship between doctors and patients is changing. With each passing generation, people expect to be more actively involved in making decisions that affect them. One study showed that "women, more educated and healthier people were more likely to prefer an active role in decision making." It also concluded that "Preferences for an active role increased with age up to 45 years but then declined."[177]

So, the consultation—the interaction between the patient and the 'expert'—is more likely to resemble a coaching session. Given that people present to primary care with similar conditions, the agenda for the meeting is set by the person making the appointment. If we accept the doctor being the 'coach' Bungay Stanier's practical approach is a step forward in how we address this issue. He sets the scene in the first chapter:

> *Only 23% of people being coached thought that the coach had a significant impact on their performance or job satisfaction. Ten per cent even suggested that the coaching they were getting was having a negative effect. (Can you imagine what it would be like going into those business meetings? "I look forward to being more confused and less motivated after my coaching sessions with you.")* [179]

The book emphasises that 'coaching' is a habit and something that needs to be valued for three reasons.

1. **To avoid team members (the patients) becoming over-dependent on the coach (the doctor).**

   *Building a coaching habit will help your team be more self-sufficient by increasing their autonomy and sense of mastery by reducing your need to jump in, take over and become the bottleneck.*[178]

There's growing concern about creating or fostering over-dependence on medicine, even in the context of life-limiting conditions. There's a significant risk of breaching ethical and legal boundaries when a patient isn't given the opportunity to explore options or make a decision contrary to the recommendations or preferred choices of their medical advisor.[179]

2. **To avoid getting overwhelmed.**

   *Building a coaching habit will help you regain focus so you and your team can do the work that has real impact and so you can direct your time, energy and resources to solve the challenges that make a difference.*[179]

   Being overwhelmed by demanding professional interactions is a known problem for doctors. It may be helpful for them to adopt an attitude where they know the patient must determine the best way forward after the consultation.[180]

3. **To help people do more work that has impact and meaning.**

   Coaching can:

   - provide the courage to step out beyond the comfortable and familiar
   - help patients assimilate from their experiences
   - literally and metaphorically increase and help fulfil her potential

   Again, this has strong resonance in healthcare, especially when the limited predictive value of tests means a positive result doesn't necessarily confirm a diagnosis. There's often considerable residual uncertainty when people seek help. Bungay Stanier's coaching habit emphasises this aspect as inherent to the interaction between coach and mentee.

Similarly, a given treatment may need to be offered to many so one person with the condition can benefit. In many cases the patient won't benefit from every available option. Sometimes they won't benefit from *any* of them.

Being able to explore the uncertainty about treatment outcomes while interacting with their doctor means the limitations of medicine can be shared rather than being shouldered solely by the practitioner.

*The Coaching Habit* prescribes asking seven questions in a specific order. The first question, which Bungay Stanier calls "the kickstart question" is arguably the most important: "What's on your mind?" Following this question by silence encourages disclosure of what's really bothering the patient.

Bungay Stanier frames it this way:

> *Because it's open, it invites people to get to the heart of the matter and share what's important to them. You're not telling them or guiding them. You're showing them trust and granting them autonomy to make choices for themselves. And yet the question is focused, too. It's not an invitation to tell you anything or everything. It's encouragement to go right away to what's exciting, what's provoking anxiety, what's all-consuming, what's waking them at 4 a.m., what's got their hearts beating fast.[181]*

Before visiting the doctor, Joanna probably discussed her issue with friends and family and formed ideas about the treatment she might need. Chances are the doctor wasn't part of that conversation and so won't know the full context of why Joanna has become ill. Even if the doctor was part of the conversation, they may not attend that specific practice on that specific day.[182]

Joanna's symptoms may affect her when she's already contending with other problems—an unhappy relationship, an unsatisfactory job, debts or other things considered 'normal.' Substance abuse is a common challenge, typically involving alcohol but sometimes illicit drugs or even prescribed drugs. These consultations are the most difficult, as Joanna may hope (or even insist) that the doctor simply issue a prescription or order a test because that's what she thinks she needs.[183]

Sometimes the problem is deeply hidden—domestic violence, child or elder abuse or some other illegal activity. These contexts may never be established as the backdrop to the patient's problems.

Similarly, doctors may not know Mick can't read or write, or that he has a questionable understanding of his own anatomy. They may even believe his symptoms are caused by something that's anatomically or physiologically impossible.[184]

A more recent problem relates to the availability of unfiltered information online. White and Horvitz define *cyberchondria* as "the unfounded escalation of concerns about common symptomatology, based on the review of search results and literature on the web."[185] A patient may misinterpret symptoms of a minor illness as something much more serious. Without exploring these ideas and concerns in detail, the doctor and the patient may never see eye to eye on an issue or understand the other's perspective.

In medical research, the quest to improve outcomes often focuses on technical solutions, preferably developed in labs staffed by people in white coats and funded by a big research grant. But we may also be able to change these outcomes (for better or for worse) by studying the dialogue in the offices of doctors' clinics.

A key principle of medical ethics is beneficence, which is described as:

> *A moral obligation to act for the benefit of others. Not all acts of beneficence are obligatory, but a principle of beneficence asserts an obligation to help others further their interests. Obligations to confer benefits, to prevent and remove harms, and to weigh and balance the possible goods against the costs and possible harms of an action are central to bioethics.*[186]

Beneficence dictates that we give autonomous individuals options that are in their best interests. That may include an operation, pills, a referral or a test. But we also need to tell them when these options will not promote their wellbeing. Robert Cialdini's book *Pre-Suasion* reviews the evidence that words predict outcomes and he strikes a note of caution in this regard:

> *Those that use the pre-suasive approach must decide what to present immediately before their message. But they must also have to make an even earlier*

> *decision: whether, on ethical grounds, to employ such*
> *an approach.*[187]

This model acknowledges the enormous power of language (for good or for ill) in the consultation. Cialdini offers four key lessons:

1. **There are 'Privileged Moments.'** Doctors should make sure the patient has been primed before the interaction to increase or diminish the impact of what they hear. We can predict what these moments might be for people in healthcare: pregnancy, being diagnosed with a significant illness, receiving worrying test results, a significant birthday, etc.

2. **The preamble to a question can sway the patient's response to be what the questioner is hoping for.** For example, the question "Given the recent cases of death from influenza, how dangerous do you perceive the threat of flu to be?" is loaded with pre-suasion. By reminding the patient about these deaths, the questioner is drawing attention to the immediacy of the topic. The patient may then evaluate the danger as high and be more likely to accept the offer of vaccination. Of course, this assumes vaccination is in her best interest and that she understands there's no guarantee the vaccine will protect her against the flu.

3. **We think whatever grabs our attention is relevant.** In other words, patients are far more likely to pay attention to and be influenced by stimuli that fit their goal in that situation. In medicine, receiving information

that suggests we might be 'at risk' of an illness might compel us to act. However, the heightened anxiety of such a message (e.g. describing bowel symptoms as early signs of cancer) can also have detrimental effects. For example, it could have driven Tegan to cling to questionable ideas about her bouts of diarrhoea during pregnancy to stifle concerns generated by the psychological threat of having cancer.

4. **It isn't just about the facts.** It's also about how they're presented. There are ways to engage (if not bypass) logic. As suggested earlier, the three most effective 'commanders' of attention are sex, threats and novelty. When an issue is presented in the context of these considerations, its effect is boosted significantly. As Cialdini puts it:

*The communicator who can fasten an audience's focus onto the favourable elements of an argument raises the chance that the argument will go unchallenged by opposing points of view, which get locked out of the attentional environment as a consequence.*[188]

We also know people have a poor understanding of numbers. Yet so much of what doctors say in the consult is couched in numeric terms e.g. "The risk of diabetes is 40 per cent." In a study of laypersons published in Health Expectations, the authors concluded that:

*Most participants thought of risk not as a neutral statistical concept, but as signifying danger and emotional threat, and viewed cancer risk in terms*

*of concrete risk factors rather than mathematical*
*probabilities. Participants had difficulty*
*acknowledging uncertainty implicit to the concept*
*of risk, and judging the statistical significance of*
*individualised risk estimates.*[189]

Patients consult doctors every day and the words used in consultations are powerful because they have influence. The most important job in healthcare is to make the patient more likely to stop smoking, eat only what they need, exercise more, get screened for an increasingly long list of diseases and actively manage their illnesses or conditions. So, the role of language in medicine isn't just to express or describe, but also to achieve these outcomes. It is done by signposting patients to form mental associations between the doctor's advice and the best possible outcomes for them.

The business of medicine isn't that different from other forms of commerce where someone offers a possible solution to a client's problem. From studying human interactions we've learned that what is said and how and when the issues are framed, can have a crucial impact on what the patient does after the interaction.

This connection is also forged by what people see and in the symbolism of what's on display when they visit a doctor.

The so-called props.

# 9

# THE PROPS

When Suzy seeks medical attention, she may be conveying "I'm unhappy," "I'm worried," "I'm bored," "I'm ashamed," "I'm tired," or "I'm not coping and these symptoms are the last straw."

With spiralling costs and growing shortages, the future of healthcare warrants a renewed commitment to the art of doctoring. It boils down to simple, cost-free choices already available to healthcare practitioners. Anything that helps the patient reveal things they feel are too embarrassing, worrying or shocking to confide in with anyone else.

The connection is also enhanced by what's on display when the patient visits a doctor. When they're distressed or worried, patients have a deep-seated need to believe a doctor can make her better. The 'medicine man' is therefore a social construct. The doctor needs to be 'special' and it must be evident throughout the encounter. Having a cluttered environment that has the health practitioner glancing at a computer screen and being distracted by paperwork, bleeping devices and flashing lights isn't conducive to sustaining the magic.

Specifically arranged furniture is a feature of most consulting rooms. A stethoscope has also been shown to increase trustworthiness in the person wearing it, even before the actors begin the drama. How the furniture is arranged can affect how a patient feels about being in that space. We know that posture, eye contact and verbal communication matter. The way a room is arranged can also emphasise the role of one person above others in that room, or alternately convey a commitment to partnership.

Research has also shown that scent has a strong effect on the quality of interactions between people in a public space. But the smell of a room is rarely considered in healthcare environments.

Of all the assets available to doctors when trying to communicate with their patients, touch is the most potent of all. Rather than get the patient onto the examination table, the doctor may request a test instead. In reality, negative or unequivocal tests lead to a spiral of further unreliable tests and increasing costs, heightening the risk of harm and over-servicing.

The benefit a patient receives from being examined with a stethoscope can go beyond the slight improvement in diagnostic accuracy from its use. When deployed in the context of a medical consultation, even the humble and inexpensive tongue depressor can help forge a relationship that makes the patient feel comfortable to reveal the real cause of their worries.

Props don't need to be high-tech or expensive but they do need to be included and used in the art of doctoring.

In his TEDx talk Fred Lee, vice-president at two major medical centres and a cast member at Walt Disney World in Florida, suggests we should focus on 'patient experience' rather than 'patient satisfaction.'[190] Therefore, doctors must be strongly encouraged to redirect the focus away from the limitations of 'patient satisfaction.'

As a clinician, I noticed by accident that when I offered Frank my high-backed leather chair and sat in the lower 'bucket seat' intended for patients, he was more likely to shake my hand as he left. This symbolic gesture often indicated that he'd had a good experience, even though I hadn't changed anything else about the way I practiced medicine. I may need to reconsider other aspects of the way I practice the art of doctoring. That simple change in the rituals of consulting had a startling result.

From that point on I swapped the seats around in my consulting room, changing how both my patients and I felt about the consult.[191] I rediscovered the value of a key prop in my room—a choice that was simple and free.

In other parts of the world, specifically in North America, there may not be much difference in the size of the chairs each 'actor' occupies. There may be other ways to make the patient feel like the most important in the room. It just needs the creativity and ingenuity of those who work in that environment to determine what they might be.

The consultation ritual includes the greeting, the exchange and the management plan. The experience is replete with icons and symbolism, which all affect the outcome. In primary care, it's unlikely that Dave will need any laboratory tests before treatment is offered. Most people present with self-limiting, short-lived and relatively benign minor illnesses.

But doctors also rely heavily on what they're told by their patients and what they might find during an examination. So, the theatre that is the consultation can't have the ambience of an accountant's office or government clerk's cubicle. If it does, patients like Suzy will react as if they're visiting a technician rather than seeking solace, advice or an opportunity to voice their distress. Joe needs 'to be seen' while his doctor craves trust and confidence. These two individuals both have needs and if neither is satisfied then the encounter will be disappointing for everyone involved.

It could be very different and in some cases it already is.

The 'medicine man' is a social construct. The first and arguably most successful doctor ever, Imhotep of ancient Egypt, didn't prescribe antibiotics or order X-rays or scans. In fact, it's his treatments were more than likely placebos.

We can consider ways clinicians can communicate their value by reflecting on how other sectors allow their customers or clients to feel safe, secure and able to be vulnerable, so they make (or consider making) radical choices. All five senses must be engaged so the patient processes and interprets the information as being a unique, memorable and valuable experience.

## The look

What Pauline and Mick crave most of all is their doctor's undivided attention. They need to believe that while they're in that doctor's presence, the doctor is wholly focused on them. A cluttered environment that has the service provider constantly glancing at a computer and being distracted by paperwork and bleeping, buzzing or flashing lights on phones or computers, isn't conducive to that feeling.

What's presented for view in the room is critically important. It includes the room itself, the associated paraphernalia and the appearance of the doctor. The furniture and the way it's arranged can have a significant impact. Clearly there needs to be:

- a range of ergonomically arranged equipment, including whatever the doctor uses to write on
- a computer
- a phone
- a couch or whatever the patient lies on during an examination
- seats
- instruments

However, those objects can be strategically deployed for best results. How positioning chairs in relation to each other can affect the room's occupants has been extensively researched. The arrangement can enhance the role of one person above all others or convey partnership.

Patients usually present with ideas about what is or isn't negotiable. They are best placed to determine the outcome of the consultation because, in the end, they must determine what's in their best interests. If the arrangement demotes the patient, the encounter is already set to be unsatisfactory at best and confrontational at worst.

In some cases, the doctor may have to deny a patient's request if they or the law deem it inappropriate. But even in those circumstances, the patient still needs to feel they've had their needs addressed and haven't been:

- subjected to discrimination
- harshly judged
- summarily dismissed from a place that looks and behaves like a government bureaucracy

The way a provider chooses to present themselves conveys something to the patient. Specific types of medical equipment can have a significant impact on how a doctor is perceived before they even speak. Displaying a stethoscope and other items has been shown to affect how trustworthy, honest, moral and genuine a doctor is considered, even before the interaction begins.[192] So it's important for doctors to display this equipment prominently, particularly the stethoscope. They should also remove clutter and organise the space so it's less distracting.

What's on display includes what the doctor is wearing. In this regard there's conflicting evidence. Some researchers don't believe it makes a difference. Others argue it depends on the observer—Pauline might prefer the doctor to be wearing more formal attire while Joe might not. Dressing smartly won't always impress the patient. It's unlikely to offend them, whereas wearing shorts or jeans might be regarded as being disrespectful.

Body language is even more critical. Patients notice where the doctor gazes during the consultation. Do they make eye contact? Do they spend their time looking at a computer screen? How do they handle their equipment?

Most consulting rooms have at least some furniture and the way it's arranged can affect how patients feel about being in that space. We know posture, eye contact and verbal communication matter.[193] We should also consider where the doctor sits in the room and even what they sit on. It's particularly relevant in boardrooms, but it also applies in any room where only two people are talking.[194]

Three factors influence perceived status and power in terms of chairs:

- the size of the chair and its accessories
- the height of the chair from the floor
- the location of the chair relative to the other person

Doctors in many countries choose to sit in executive chairs, which convey authority.[195] (The fact they're comfortable may also be relevant.) Nevertheless, they create an impression that whoever's using them has alpha status in the room.[196] Evidence suggests the way doctors position themselves relative to the patient matters in any setting—office or ward.[197]

Doctors need to create the impression they're spending more time with their patients, because in some cases there's no more time available. Doctors can't do much about healthcare policy or resourcing, at least not in the short term. However, by changing the consulting room's seating arrangements they can give patients the impression they're more present and therefore providing a longer and more satisfying consult.

## The smell

Is there a smell you associate with your doctor's clinic? If there is, it's probably not a pleasant one.

I remember the waiting room of my childhood doctor. He consulted from his home (as most doctors did at the time) and patients waited in his converted garage. It was always cold and smelled damp—not a nice place to be when you had a fever or were anticipating an injection. The unpleasant memories of being ill and expecting pain were linked to the musty smell of that waiting room.

Researchers document similar trends:

> *Subjects then rated their memories as to how happy or unhappy the events recalled were at the time they occurred. Subjects in the pleasant odour condition produced a significantly higher percentage of happy memories than did subjects in the unpleasant odour condition. When subjects who did not find the odours at least moderately pleasant or unpleasant were removed from the analysis, more pronounced effects on memory were found.[198]*

*Fortune* made a similar point in non-medical contexts:

> *Still, many companies are seeking to develop experiences that go a bit beyond a phone or a computer—a fact that isn't lost on Fabrigas. "We spend so much time, money, and energy on crafting our logo and doing our color palette and picking our music and the uniform of our hospitality staff," she says. "But the scent is the thing that really wraps all of that together.*

*It's almost like your logo in the air".[199]*

Of all the ways healthcare providers can tailor the experience they offer; smell is potentially the most powerful. While they may carefully select the colour scheme, the magazines and even the floor coverings and video entertainment, they rarely consider choosing a smell. Perhaps it's because humans were thought to have a poor sense of smell until relatively recently. Research has since debunked that myth:

> *These results indicate that humans are not poor smellers (a condition technically called microsmats), but instead are relatively good, perhaps even excellent, smellers (macrosmats). This may come as a surprise to many people, though not to those who make their living by their noses, such as oenologists, perfumers, and food scientists. Anyone who has taken part in a wine tasting, or observed professional testing of food flavours or perfumes, knows that the human sense of smell has extraordinary capacities for discrimination.[200]*

Here's *Fortune* again:

> *We tend to remember moments in our lives based on how we lived them across our five senses. Companies dealing with declining sales and rising rents are trying to diversify ways to appeal to those five senses, hoping to draw in more customers and actually shape the way they live and breathe the brand by evoking certain sensations.[201]*

Research has consistently shown that scent has an essential effect not only on satisfaction, but also on the quality of the interactions between people in a public space. This has implications for the value of one of the consultation's 'props'— the smell.

Patient experience is about engaging them with all five senses. Some service providers are already onto this.[202] Many providers and retailers pump out specific scents in their premises or on aeroplanes as a signature of their brand. In those instances, you're likely to associate the brand with that scent and it creates a strong positive memory that's invoked every time you walk into those premises or board that aircraft.

## The feel

Possibly the most crucial aspect of the healthcare experience is the physical contact associated with a visit to a doctor.

Of all the assets available to doctors in their attempts to communicate with patients, touch is the most important of all. Few other service providers can leverage this sense. Those who can (e.g. hairdressers, masseurs, manicurists) are thriving. As society changes, people are unlikely to experience touch as often as they need. People now spend more time in the virtual world than in physical contact.[203]

Being touched when feeling unwell, vulnerable and distressed satisfies a deep emotional need. Yet in the haste to move patients through their clinic, doctors now examine people less often than was custom and practice a few decades ago.

At the same time, technology improvements have created more sophisticated tests. So, doctors may be more inclined to order tests than rely on clinical acumen to make a diagnosis. Nonetheless, there's a therapeutic aspect to consultations that isn't being addressed because doctors are limiting themselves in the pursuit of quantifiable data.

It's been suggested that many aspects of the examination are neither sensitive nor specific and so the positive predictive value of the physical findings are modest.[204] For example, that icon of medicine the stethoscope offers limited information and in many cases may not be serviced regularly to maintain its limited value. However, Suzy may crave the ritual of an examination involving the stethoscope more than the slight increase in diagnostic accuracy. In no other circumstance would Suzy allow another person (and a stranger to boot) to apply a metal disc to her bare chest, let alone view and palpate her bare abdomen or examine her intimately. In this setting, the patient can feel both vulnerable and safe.

The intimacy and symbolic value of the examination forges a strong psychological connection between doctor and patient. Unfortunately, opportunities to forge this connection are increasingly jettisoned in favour of impersonal tests, even though they're unlikely to aid diagnosis.

An otherwise healthy and young patient presenting with fatigue is unlikely to be sick. However, after considering the time it would take for the patient to undress and climb onto the examination table, the doctor may request a test instead. In this context the test is unlikely to aid treatment. It may even do harm by creating the expectation that tests are the most important tools in medicine rather than words or touch.

In reality, negative or unequivocal tests in light of persistent symptoms lead to a spiral of further tests and increasing costs, as well as a higher risk of harming patients and over-servicing. So, to increase the value of the medical consultation, most if not all people who see a doctor needs to experience touch.

## Taste

Of the five senses, the one patients are least likely to associate with a visit to the doctor is taste.

Most prescribed medicines (especially the liquid variety) have a taste.[205] Many other industries use taste to enhance their abilities to connect potential customers to their products. This is obviously true in the food industry, where the taste of food is carefully crafted to release dopamine at the very thought of it.[206]

But there's one medical innovation that's more likely to yield a diagnosis than an X-ray. What's more, it's available worldwide, is cheaper than the cheapest stethoscope and requires less training to operate than a tendon hammer.

What is it? A tongue depressor.

And why is more likely to yield a diagnosis? Because when deployed within the context of a medical consultation— when the practitioner is giving a patient their undivided attention—the tongue depressor forges a relationship that can trigger them to express their deepest concerns. After all, in what other social context can you shove a piece of wood into someone's open mouth and get them to say "Ahh?"

A few years ago, I consulted a 50-year-old mother of five working as a supermarket checkout assistant who was complaining of a sore throat. She talked about how awful she felt and how she was struggling with her job, getting frequent bouts of tonsillitis and afraid of losing her job.

She had a mildly red throat and I thought I'd find evidence of an active infection in her neck. But her temperature was normal and I concluded that it was most likely a simple cold.

As I turned around to put the tongue depressor into a bin, she burst into tears.

"There's something else I need to tell you doctor. I'm now working as a prostitute because for the first time in 10 years I haven't been able to afford my kids' schoolbooks."

It's the last thing I expected to hear. And it certainly wasn't something medical school taught me could result from examining a throat. It's one of the myriad of reasons general practice is the most challenging medical specialty. Nothing is necessarily what it seems.

Needless to say, our consultation took a very different direction. She was screened for other infections and fortunately the tests were negative. We then talked about her dilemma and she decided there may be better ways to furnish her kids with what they needed for school.

There's little evidence to suggest examining the throat can aid diagnosis in most cases. Penicillin doesn't hasten recovery even when it is targeting the right bugs. But anyone with a sore throat who consults a doctor expects to be examined. Otherwise, why would people seek medical advice about a cold? It's common knowledge that in most cases the only effective treatment is rest, fluids and regular doses of paracetamol.

When a patient presents with a minor self-limiting illness, they're often expressing concern about some other aspect of their life.[207] If the healthcare professional is receptive they may 'hear' the patient telling them, "I'm unhappy," "I'm worried," "I'm bored," "I'm feeling guilty," "I'm tired" or "I'm not coping and this discomfort is the last straw."

There are tools we seldom do without. A stethoscope is vital and not just because of what the doctor hears when they put it to the chest. Props don't need to be high-tech or expensive—a tongue depressor costs 13 cents. In the right hands, such simple equipment can be extraordinarily powerful.

# 10

# THE ACTION

A key factor in the Theatre Model© is what happens when the patients are in the consulting room.

For a start it's a question of who they see. If Pauline and Mick choose to see a different doctor every time (as would be their right in many countries), that doesn't necessarily mean they're choosing or receiving inferior care.

Policymakers may be tempted to deploy financial incentives to drive efficiencies or hit targets and as part of that strategy force people to visit the same doctor every time. Such incentives can be deployed as a weapon, forcing medical professionals to do the bidding of politicians and bureaucrats.

It's short-sighted (not to mention naïve) to think incentives are enough to deliver better health and reduce costs. Such incentives assume that patients behave rationally and that easy fixes can be quickly delivered on a prescription pad or by ordering tests.

Such ideas are also promoted by commercial interests that profit from products or services with limited research evidence but superb marketing. (Pills that treat obesity are a classic example.) Clinical protocols have also promoted expensive solutions that did more harm than good, as was the case for prescriptions of some long-term medications many years ago.

The other side of the coin is that family doctors are expected to ration care, by authorising it according to criteria determined by 'experts.' Effective healthcare solutions can't rely on the options that could be open to interpretation. Effective innovations only trigger people to do what they already want to do.

The best solutions are enthusiastically embraced and adopted by their target audiences, which in healthcare includes the doctors. Behind the 'big data' of over-servicing lurks the stories of ineffective consultations where:

- the patient isn't examined
- the doctor takes an incomplete history
- the risks and benefits aren't explained in a way that leads to better decisions

Why else would a patient at negligible risk of malignancy willingly choose to have invasive instrumental examinations of their private parts?

The most effective route to better outcomes is to promote the art of doctoring.

---

All the patients I've described will consult a doctor in the course of a typical year. They're also likely to visit a pharmacy and/or seek advice from a pharmacist. Some will go to an outpatient clinic and a few will spend time in a hospital.[208]

Of those who go to see a doctor, some patients will consult the same doctor they saw previously. Other patients (e.g. Joe and Jonathan) may visit the same practice but not necessarily the same doctor. A significant number of people will visit more than one practice.

One strategy is to force patients to see the same doctor or the same practice by restructuring payments rather than having a 'fee for service' where they can go to any clinic. Another is to introduce electronic health records that follow them through the various providers they choose to consult.

The latter idea is fraught with adverse privacy implications (not to mention technical challenges) and has been effectively introduced in very few countries. The former is politically challenging. For example, in the UK payments were eventually linked to clinical performance targets as part of the government's desire to control healthcare costs. As a result, the focus shifted to what could be measured as if that's all that mattered.

Whatever the rhetoric, there's a temptation to deploy financial incentives to drive efficiency or reach targets. Some argue they're the most effective incentives that can be weaponised, forcing a profession to act on the whims of politicians and bureaucrats.

People assume that continuity of care is a good thing. On that basis, a patient who consults the same doctor every time will have better health. Most of us have a relative who will insist on seeing the same doctor every time.

"No one but Dr Smith will do," Aunt Kate tells you sternly.

But Dr Smith has some 'interesting' approaches to Aunt Kate's problems. Despite knowing her for years, Dr Smith hasn't worked out that her latest symptoms could be a manifestation of some family drama. For example, she might suddenly be more bothered about her aching hip because Uncle John is making her miserable, or because he's making her carry the shopping across the car park when they go to the mall on Friday evening.

So is there strong evidence that a patient who consults the same doctor every time will be:

- Less likely to be prescribed inappropriate drugs or unnecessary tests? Maybe.[209]
- More likely to have symptoms of cancer recognised early? Not really.[210]
- More likely to be counselled about poor lifestyle choices? Maybe.[211]
- More likely to be screened for long-term illness? Maybe.[212]
- More likely to be protected from infectious diseases? Maybe.[213]
- More likely to have better outcomes from long-term illness? Maybe.[214]

The evidence is equivocal at best. Even the most ardent supporters of continuity conclude there is "lots more research needed". It suggests that choosing to see different doctors doesn't necessarily mean the patient is choosing or receiving inferior care.

The metric that healthcare is usually judged on relates to whether the sector can prevent the demise of a patient from a life-limiting illness or reduce morbidity from a long-term illness. For a politician, nothing is more compelling than numbers that prove their policies work. Understandably there's an incentive to persuade, motivate or otherwise coerce clinicians to 'follow guidelines,' as if that alone will deliver the best outcomes for patients and therefore reduce costs.

Some commentators believe that if doctors did what the bureaucrats tell them to then everything would be fine, as demonstrated by graphs on a spreadsheet. They rely on the assumption that a patient always behaves rationally and that easy fixes can be delivered on a prescription pad or by ordering a test.

More often than not, they're also promoted by commercial interests that profit considerably from products or services with little or no research evidence but superb marketing.

In the past some doctors have prescribed:

- Hormone replacement therapy for menopause on the basis that it effectively rejuvenated the woman, despite the lack of unequivocal scientific evidence.[215]
- Antidepressants for cases of social phobia or unhappy life situations, with questionable results.[216]
- Lipid-lowering drugs for people who might benefit more from making different lifestyle choices.[217]
- Scans for stress-related headaches.[218]
- Spinal X-rays for muscular back pain.[219]
- Antibiotics for viral illness.[220]

(Some of them still do.)

There's evidence to suggest that doctors who order tests to keep the patient happy are misguided.[221]

From the funder's perspective, access to tests and specialists must be limited by cost. So, there's a belief that family doctors can and should ration care by limiting tests and treatment to urgent cases that 'merit' referral based on the views of recognised 'experts.'

Cancer is a case in point. Of course, doctors know it's not a single condition. Its biology varies, as do the responses of its victims. Tegan presented with hardly any symptoms but died within three months. Other patients have presented with a plethora of horrible complaints but had very treatable tumours.

Perhaps one day computers will identify people such as Tegan based on data routinely collected from body sensors and personal devices. That may sound wonderful, but it means Tegan's intimate data will be relayed to and stored on a machine. She may not know who else can access that information, or for what purpose. A privacy breach could have implications of Orwellian proportions.

In the meantime, one proposed 'solution' involved deploying computers that used algorithms based on evidence-based guidelines to refer 'high-risk' patients to specialists. But this 'solution' relied on:

- family doctors referring everyone who presented with 'red flag' symptom

- hospitals correctly prioritising those patients when they received the computer-generated referral

In other words, the solution assumed that when one person did X, the people in the other part of the system would do Y and the outcome would be Z.

As you can probably imagine, it didn't go well.

- Family doctors (GPs) didn't always recognise the symptom complexes touted as being the hallmarks of risk.[222]
- GPs in one experiment were reticent to deploy the software anywhere outside of simulations with actors.[223]
- Specialists didn't prioritise cases the computer identified as urgent.[224]

There's also limited evidence that people referred based on such criteria would always have better outcomes.

- Diseases such as cancer have a different impact on every individual.
- People with cancer don't always present the same way.
- Doctors may not agree with the experts, even when those 'experts' are medical practitioners.
- Doctors may decide not to take up an innovation for various reasons.
- The 'system' consists of many moving parts. For a system with seven parts, if the 'right thing' occurred 80% of the time at each step, then only 21% (0.8 x 0.8 x 0.8 x 0.8 x 0.8 x 0.8 x 0.8) of people would benefit from the 'plan.'[225]

Businesses can't rely on navigating multiple risky steps successfully. A far better idea is to trigger doctors to do what they already want to do. The best innovators work on solutions their target audiences will enthusiastically embrace and adopt. In healthcare that includes doctors.

There's plenty of evidence that 'continuity of care' increases a person's trust in a doctor, as with the earlier example involving Aunt Kate. But there's no evidence that Aunt Kate will be better off trusting her doctor because trust (which isn't consistently defined[226]) doesn't guarantee better outcomes. If Aunt Kate visits her GP with symptoms of bone cancer and is referred for urgent investigation because the doctor recognised the clinical signs, then she will have been well served regardless of whom she sees or where.

The point is that one of them should practice the art of doctoring and spot what's out of the ordinary.[227]

## The interaction is key

In 2017, an 80-year-old woman (let's call her Catherine) fell to the ground on a pavement and waited for 14 hours to be seen in the emergency department of a major city hospital. Bruised from head to toe, she was 'triaged' and then moved back into the crowded emergency waiting room.

She was examined by a medical student and briefly by a doctor, who recorded that any deterioration in her vision as a result of a bleed into her brain couldn't be assessed because she didn't have her glasses.

Given she seemed otherwise well, she was sent home with her granddaughter and asked to return a couple of days later.

And when she did, she had to wait another nine hours for another check.

Is this the kind of care any healthcare system should deliver?

If you're a doctor, what's it like to be *your* patient? Ask yourself:

- Why do patients visit you and not some other doctor practising nearby?
- How long do your patients wait?
- How are they greeted on arrival?
- What do they do while they wait and how do they feel about waiting?
- How long do they see you, on average?
- What can they expect from the visit?
- When do you order tests and why? What difference do these tests make to the outcome?
- Why do you prescribe those drugs? How many people take them as prescribed?
- Why do you ask them to return for a follow-up appointment?
- When and why do you refer them to someone else?
- What do they tell their family about your service?

No business would survive without a thorough understanding of this information.

Catherine had to go to a government funded hospital emergency department because she could have had a life-threatening injury. In the hospital's defence the manager might say that given the resources available it had no option but to offer the service as described. But where is the data to demonstrate it was the lack of options rather than a lack of thought in organising one of its most essential services?

When it comes to life-saving treatments, hospitals will probably maintain their monopoly for some time. But what about family medicine? There may be scope for this kind of service to be provided by someone who is just as qualified, will see her much sooner and will offer her a cup of tea while she waits for the X-rays to be reported. What scope is there to provide better care than what doctors currently provide? What effect could this have on other healthcare providers?

William Barnett is credited with this prediction:

> *A newer take on the organisational environment is the "Red Queen" theory, which highlights the relative nature of progress. The theory is borrowed from ecology's Red Queen hypothesis that successful adaptation in one species is tantamount to a worsening environment for others, which must adapt in turn to cope with the new conditions. The theory's name is inspired by the character in Lewis Carroll's Through the Looking Glass who seems to be running but is staying in the same spot. In a 1996 paper, William Barnett describes Red Queen competition among organisations as a process of mutual learning. A company is forced by direct competition to improve its performance, in turn, increases the pressure on its rivals, thus creating a virtuous circle of learning and competition.[228]*

The *Weekend Australian* headline on 24 April 2016 declared that 'Healthcare waste costs $20bn a year.' According to the graph on the first page of the article, in 2004 there were 105–110 family doctors (GPs) or specialists for every 100,000 people. While the number of GPs has remained static since then, there are now more than 130 specialists per 100,000 people. So according to the Australian Commission on Safety and Quality in Health Care, the rising cost of waste in healthcare runs parallel to the increase in specialists.[229]

Unfortunately, there's nothing new about this story. Similar trends have occurred in previous decades. According to established formulas, more primary care equals lower costs. As the late Barbara Starfield wrote:

> *Six mechanisms, alone and in combination, may account for the beneficial impact of primary care on population health. They are (1) greater access to needed services, (2) better quality of care, (3) a greater focus on prevention, (4) early management of health problems, (5) the cumulative effect of the main primary care delivery characteristics, and (6) the role of primary care in reducing unnecessary and potentially harmful specialist care.[230]*

What was disappointing was the accompanying commentary suggesting the solution is political. The journalistic analysis was that powerful lobby groups have influenced policy to the point where there's subsidised over-servicing of the population, especially for prostatectomies, colonoscopies, arthroscopies, cataract surgery, hysterectomies and CT scans.

In any country where general practice is the gatekeeper to specialist services, we need to figure out how to tackle this problem for the sake of the economy. However, we need to remain vigilant about quick fixes, as we've learnt that chasing votes rarely delivers a lasting solution.

In medicine, Frank might be referred or persuaded to have treatment or investigations. Beneath the 'big data' lurks the story of ineffective consultations—not examining the patient, taking an incomplete history or not explaining the risks and benefits of tests and treatments in a way that helps the patient make an informed decision.

After all, why else would a patient at very low risk choose to have a colonoscopy?

What's the difference between handling a request for antibiotics for a cold and one for an equally pointless CT scan for muscular back pain? When it comes to taking action when sick people turn up in doctors' clinics, the most effective solution is to practice the art of doctoring.

# CONCLUSION

Most healthcare is delivered by family doctors in clinics, not by staff in hospitals. So, it stands to reason that family medicine is where we should practice the art of doctoring most skilfully.

In the end what matters most is the perspective of the patients—not what a healthcare system provides to remain viable using proxy markers of excellence. When patients are treated like numbers, we get the unsatisfactory results we're now witnessing.

In healthcare, policymakers have favoured quantum of access over quality interactions with a skilful doctor. We need to harness the intuitions and insights of those who consult patients daily behind closed doors. In the foreseeable future, patients may only seek help when they experience symptoms. On these occasions, doctors have the opportunity to practice their art and promote decisions that improve long-term prognosis.

There's a compelling case for doctors to lead healthcare redesign. They face a challenging and uncertain future and have as much to gain from the art of doctoring as their patients. Perhaps the most significant opportunity presented to us today is the creativity of doctors and their staff. The next major advance in healthcare is likely to be crafted by people working in specific circumstances with a particular group of patients. Therefore, the redesign should focus as much on doctors as diseases.

My call to action is for doctors to create more opportunities for better human connections. In other words, to practice the art of doctoring. It starts with recognising that the patient is the most important person in the clinical encounter.

Excellence in communication is often considered quaint and irrelevant. But to improve the outcome of a consultation—one where someone like Dave (lifestyle) might respond to useful information—we must focus on the theatre and rituals within the consultation. We can no longer squander the opportunities it offers to nudge and trigger our patients to make better choices.

It seems strange that a sector with the biggest opportunity to forge intimate alliances with stakeholders sacrifices these assets to keep the commerce machine rolling. Healthcare is now a profitable business, but if we medicalise human distress, we risk losing healthcare's real value to society—making and keeping people well.

Many successful companies have outlined the recipe for creating conditions that engage customers. They're not driven by targets, employee incentives or cycling through successive chief executives. The fundamentals of business success are generated by the customer experience—especially when serving that customer is the reason the company exists in the first place.

In healthcare, that reason is to safeguard and promote health and wellbeing.

---

With reference to the Theatre Model© most healthcare premises can be reorganised with a minimum of investment—furniture rearranged, walls and shelves decluttered, old and tired equipment replaced or tidied away, walls repainted, dog-eared posters taken down, water cooler installed.

For a relatively low cost the space can made to smell nice.

But perhaps the most effective 'innovation' is the attitude of the staff, especially the doctor. Much of this can be achieved without changing policy and can benefit most people who need healthcare. It takes little effort to stand up and greet a patient, offer them a comfortable seat, make eye contact with them and let them speak freely for two minutes at the start of a meeting. Practicing the art of doctoring is far less time-consuming than dealing with the consequences of not making use of the assets it deploys.

The healthcare industry is ripe for disruption. In the absence of the art of doctoring, primary care as a business will struggle to maintain its market share. To date, researchers in primary care often fail to engage with clinicians and innovation is stymied. Government investment in research is limited and risk averse.

For example, 90% of government-funded healthcare in Australia is delivered at small clinics. Yet more than 90% of government investment in research and innovation is targeted elsewhere. The limited funding available is usually awarded to competing tertiary institutions whose performance is measured in traditional academic outputs (mainly published papers) rather than any effect on practice.[231]

To make an appreciable contribution to health, research must address real-world problems for patients. The recurring themes at academic medical research conferences have hardly changed in decades. Many projects are exploratory and despite a plethora of published research papers, hardly ever result in tangible solutions such as:

- investigating why outcomes for Pauline (pneumonia) remain poor
- exploring the needs of minority groups under-served by the healthcare system
- engaging doctors to help Joe (obesity) eat less, drink less and exercise more
- working out what's wrong with people like Fran (headaches) who visit doctors more often than average
- defining the characteristics of people like Tegan (cancer) who need healthcare sooner
- identifying the key performance indicators so doctors can receive suitable financial incentives
- surveying or interviewing doctors about their patients or their work

- getting healthcare professionals from different disciplines working together to benefit patients such as Angela (home visit) with complex unmet needs under the leadership of a medical practitioner
- developing tools to research all of the above

Perhaps it's time to swap these themes for an alternative set of projects more specifically targeted to generating tangible solutions including:

- how to trigger lifestyle behaviour change when patients are ready to change, rather than promoting medication or surgery as the means to arrive at best results
- what needs to be done when and by whom to get Pauline (pneumonia) what she needs when the need is urgent
- how to signpost Jonathan (tests), Frank (snoring) and Fran (headaches) to more appropriate sources of advice
- how to share the decision making with Frank (snoring), considering the limited benefits and appreciable risks of drugs and surgery
- what can be achieved when health practitioners focus on what they're good at rather than being distracted by issues beyond their interest, training or expertise and stop them trying to solve problems with pills
- look more closely at how doctors and patients interact rather than just what's recorded and find specific ways to promote whatever benefits Frank in specific circumstances

The next significant advance in healthcare is likely to be crafted piecemeal and focus as much on doctors as diseases. Here's Paul Graham:

> *The way you'll get big ideas in, say, health care is by starting out with small ideas. If you try to do some big thing, you don't just need it to be big; you need it to be good. And it's really hard to do big and good simultaneously. So, what that means is you can either do something small and good and then gradually make it bigger, or do something big and bad and gradually make it better. And you know what? Empirically, starting big just does not work. That's the way the government does things. They do something really big that's really bad, and they think, Well, we'll make it better, and then it never gets better.[232]*

These issues, like the art of doctoring, speak to the heart of what we consider professionalism in healthcare. And while you'll find little consensus on this issue in the literature, commentators acknowledge that doctor is as doctor does:

> *Medical professionalism is exemplified through what physicians actually do—how they meet their responsibilities to individual patients and to communities. Any definition must, therefore, be clearly grounded in the nature of the physician's work. The values and behaviours that individual physicians demonstrate in their daily interactions with patients and their families, and with physicians and other professional colleagues, become the foundation on which medical professionalism rests.[233]*

Nine behaviours are identified as the hallmark of professionalism in medicine. Among them are some I've highlighted as important in the art of doctoring:

> *Honesty and integrity, caring and compassion, altruism and empathy, respect for others, and trustworthiness. Some might argue that humanistic values are not requisite to professional behaviour, that a physician can exemplify professionalism without humanism. Yet values such as compassion, altruism, integrity, and trustworthiness are so central to the nature of the physician's work, no matter what form that work takes, that no physician can indeed be effective without holding deeply such values.*[235]

By disengaging the creativity of doctors and their staff, we're losing the opportunity to truly heal people. What doctors crave most is the confidence and trust of their patients. This is within their grasp and not necessarily driven by a monetary reward.

The focus to date has been on accessing doctors to more of the same: quantity rather than quality. But within existing resources, physicians can still achieve greater job satisfaction. To reduce complaints and increase patient confidence and trust in their abilities, doctors must boost their connection with them.

It's the reason most gifted and creative young people enter the medical profession in the first place.

The single most frequent reason for conflict between doctors and patients is lack of communication. To overcome that failure, we must recast the role of the doctor. Instead of being a technician or bureaucrat peddling procedures and products, they need to become a healer and advocate who can potentially prevent a patient putting their wellbeing at risk.

Family medicine in Australia is a private business. There are 7,200 small clinics in Australia generating $10 billion in revenue annually. Ninety-five percent of the income for these businesses is derived from government rebates, mostly from 10- to 15-minute consultations. In this context, the practitioners' main concerns are said to be:

- threat of litigation
- too much work to do in a limited time
- not earning enough money
- patients who are difficult to manage
- paperwork
- intrusion of work on family life
- the cost of practice overheads
- time pressure to see patients
- unrealistic community expectations
- negative media comments

Increases in the government rebates have failed to keep pace with the costs of running services. The shortfall is often made up by increasing patient throughput. In these circumstances, it may not be possible to offer patients additional advice or services beyond their immediate needs.

According to one study:

*Under the central set of assumptions used in*
*this study, total health and residential aged care*
*expenditure is projected to increase by 189% in*
*the period 2003 to 2033 from $85 billion to $246*
*billion—an increase of $161 billion... This is an*
*increase from 9.3% of gross domestic product (GDP)*
*in 2002–03 to 12.4% in 2032–33. Increases in the*
*volume of services per treated case are projected to*
*account for half of this increase (50%).*[234]

We know the healthcare needs of patients are set to change in three important ways:

1.  The population is aging.
2.  More effective (but also more expensive) treatments are available.
3.  Poor lifestyle choices, (especially those resulting in obesity) will generate greater demand for medical services.

We're relying on private businesses to respond to these growing needs, despite the fact they're already working to capacity. To that end, I endorse three foundations for a lean, agile and creative approach to innovation based on commercial reality:

1.  The most expensive component of innovation is establishing the problem and creating a value proposition that factors in the perspective of end users.[235]

2. Innovation only ever works when it's driven by champions willing and able to re-engineer multiple prototypes to solve the problem.

3. There are opportunities for commercial partnerships if the key performance is reframed in the metrics of sales.

The conditions for this innovative approach to family medicine already exist. However, the potential to improve outcomes for patients has been problematic because the people best placed to achieve those outcomes (the doctors) aren't directly engaged in driving reform.

The lessons I learnt from Suzy, Frank, Dave and the other cases I've presented in this book can be summarised in the rituals I now deploy as the art of doctoring.

Let's imagine Georgia is waiting in a primary care clinic.

*She's been ignoring a pain in her side for weeks, hoping it would just go away. There's too much else for her to deal with. Her partner Josh lost his job last week. Her mother had a stroke three weeks ago. Her dad is barely coping with caring for his disabled wife.*

*The children are going to a new school and Emily (nine) is having trouble settling into the new class. Georgia was hoping for a promotion at the office. With Josh out of work they certainly need the money. And it looks like Georgia might need to spend her weekends helping her dad manage at home.*

*The pain has gotten steadily worse and now it's disturbing her at night. She mentioned it to her friend who bullied her into making this appointment.*

*Georgia doesn't know her doctor well. She just
wants this nightmare to end. She thinks it might be
a urinary tract infection, but surely that wouldn't
last weeks. She doesn't want to think about the other
possibilities.*

*She didn't tell Josh she was coming to the clinic today,
giving him the impression she needed to come to this
end of town to collect something for work. She doesn't
want Josh to worry, even though he may have noticed
her holding her side while making the children's
lunches last night.*

*"Please let it be a urinary tract infection so a course of
antibiotics will fix it," she whispers to herself.*

*Georgia can't handle any more bad news. All she's
expecting is a quick visit and a prescription.*

Some healthcare clinics operate as if the doctor's time
is more important than the patient's. In most industries,
providers go above and beyond to ensure their business revolves
around the needs of the customer. Every touch point—from
the design of the building to the floor coverings—is carefully
determined. The skills and training of the frontline staff are
honed to ensure every customer feels valued and welcomed.
What the customer sees, smells, feels and hears throughout
their visit are all carefully considered. The entire experience is
choreographed and nothing is left to chance.

Preparation for Georgia's meeting with the doctor should
begin before the clinic's staff come to work. Everyone who
interacts with patients should be well rested and they should

be nourished and mindful as they enter the clinic. The desk (if there's one in the room) must be clean and the walls should display only information that staff would be willing to speak to any patient about.

There might be one or two personal mementos on display to let Georgia know the doctor is human—not that they have a particular political or religious affiliation. Mobile phones should be turned off while the practitioner consults their patient.

Before and after every patient (and perhaps even during the consult), the practitioner will wash their hands as mindfully as possible, so they're present for the meeting. A healthcare professional will greet Georgia, making eye contact and ensuring she and whoever came to the clinic with her knows the professional's name.

If the room is furnished with different chairs, Georgia will be offered the most comfortable seat. The professional will sit once Georgia has taken her seat and move away from any desk or other barrier once they've opened Georgia's medical record.

The practitioner will face Georgia and let her explain the reason for her visit without interruption. When she finishes speaking, the professional can ask if there's something else on Georgia's mind.

Having summarised what they've heard, they'll unpack each issue Georgia wants to discuss and clarify what she hopes to get from her visit. Outlining the context in which Georgia is seeking help is crucial at this stage. What Georgia does all day and where she spends her time is relevant. The people living with Georgia (who may be waiting to hear the outcome of her visit) must also be acknowledged.

Every patient must be examined by a doctor in some way. If the professional needs to use their computer during the visit, they'll tell Georgia they're focusing on the screen and will let her know exactly what they're recording and why.

Towards the end of the meeting, the professional will summarise their conversation and offer an opinion about what might help. If necessary, they'll show Georgia a model or picture of something to help explain their reasoning.

When the professional is sure Georgia has understood what's going on, they'll offer advice on what to do if things are still worrying her or if something happens she doesn't expect. With parents of young children and carers of older people, it's important to emphasise that changes can be both sudden and unexpected and that returning for another visit is okay.

As Georgia gets up to leave, the practitioner with her at the time should give her a farewell greeting and recap what she should do next. They will walk together to the door and the professional will wait until Georgia moves down the corridor before walking back into their room.

They will then sanitise their hands and prepare to see the next patient. That includes checking whether they need a break to clear their mind of any other distractions before repeating the rituals with the next patient.

## *Here's a consultation ritual checklist for the health professional.*

1. Greet the patient by name and introduce yourself.

2. Ensure the patient is seated before sitting down.

3. Make eye contact.

4. Do not interrupt the patient for at least two minutes.

5. Enquire about the circumstances surrounding the patient's visit, not just their symptoms.

6. Summarise the patient's account and clarify their expectations.

7. Wash or sanitise your hands.

8. Examine the patient.

9. Provide a diagnosis and explanation.

10. Explain what you are recording in the notes.

11. Advise what should prompt a revisit and who is responsible for the next steps..

12. Advise what to do if symptoms unexpectedly worsen.

13. Offer a farewell greeting and recap what the patient should do next.

14. Make sure you're ready to see the next patient.

15. Take a break if you need one.

Repeat the ritual for each patient.

Policymakers, like researchers, have the thankless job of delivering quick, measurable profitable results. In the healthcare business the current policies are in force only through the tenure of the vice president or chief executive. In this context, the most limiting factor to improving patient outcomes is the slavish devotion to:

- research and policy reform
- 'measurable' or so-called 'big data'

These metrics can be quoted to shareholders/voters, the editors of journals and the panels in grant applications. It's far easier to say more patients are being seen than to talk about improving patient engagement and empowerment. As a result, these metrics encourage short-term increases in patient throughput rather than actual improvements in health and wellbeing. After all, wellbeing is hard to quantify and therefore unlikely to attract policy investment.

What ultimately matters is the difference doctors make in the course of their work. In other words, how skilfully they practice the art of doctoring.

# TAKING ACTION

### *How can I use what this book is proposing to be a better doctor?*

The healthcare system in most countries is under enormous pressure. Resources are limited and demand is growing. Despite an unsatisfactory state of affairs, it's unlikely that any government will invest more to meet the needs of all patients.

At the same time, what's considered normal by most people is being recalibrated. The expectations of patients are being increased due to enhanced convenience and competition. We're unlikely to be offered more convenience in healthcare, even though the best outcomes depend on the quality of face-to-face encounters with patients when they're sick, distressed or worried.

So, it's important to make the most of the time available during your brief consultations. That means taking fuller account of the Theatre Model© and ensuring the conditions in which you practice the art of doctoring are optimal. It also means revisiting elements of the consultation you may have taken for granted—things that may seem obvious and simple but aren't often brought into play during the consultation.

## How will doing what you suggest make things better for patients?

We're all patients, and so everyone will benefit from the Theatre Model©.

When we're distressed or worried, interacting with the person best equipped to help in optimal conditions helps a great deal. It empowers us to disclose our concerns, no matter how irrational or embarrassing they might be. It makes us feel we've been seen and heard despite the relatively short visit.

The context in which we've developed symptoms (which is often pathogenic and yet considered normal) is considered and that the health professional can trigger our best efforts to improve our prognosis.

## How can doctors feel/be convinced these small changes can make a difference despite the pressures of the current healthcare environment?

There's ample evidence to support for each important factor in the Theatre Model©. Some comes from medical research and some comes from other disciplines. The best evidence comes from what we experience as reality.

In this book I mention only things I believe are within the scope of any doctor or health professional to deliver. They don't require any major changes to policy. I did this deliberately because I don't think any major investment in healthcare will happen any time soon.

Nevertheless, we urgently need outcomes to improve. Doctors are getting used to having their results presented as data:

- the proportion of people who make quantifiable changes in their health risks
- the number of people referred for unnecessary tests
- the number of medications and referrals offered

Equally important is how doctors feel during a lifelong career of selflessly serving those who need their help. If it's good for patients, it must also be good for doctors.

Because in the Theatre Model© both actors—the doctor and their patient—must experience a happy ending.

# ACKNOWLEDGEMENTS

I want to start by thanking the many patients who have trusted me to be their doctor over the past 30 years.

I also want to acknowledge three great teachers, my first ever senior nursing colleague Eileen Dorley, my high school teacher Patrick O'Sullivan and the late Prof James McCormack, professor of community medicine at Trinity College Dublin. They will likely never know the impact they had on my life and career.

I hope my description of Eileen Dorley's role during my first days on the hospital wards demonstrates how much it meant to have an experienced colleague help me make the transition from student to doctor.

Patrick O'Sullivan or POS as he was known to us from our report cards, was a legendary maths teacher. POS taught us to think clearly, to enjoy solving problems and to be tenacious. With his dark-rimmed spectacles and signature blue corduroy jacket with a hint of chalk dust on his sleeve, POS made an impression on every student he taught. He got the best out of his teenage students not by raising his voice but merely by expressing genuine concern. I wouldn't have earned a place in medical school without his help.

James McCormack was similarly a giant among his peers. He held our rapt attention by removing his glass eye to clean it during lectures. Well before the era of fake news, he pointed out that research and epidemiology can be manipulated to the detriment of patients. He introduced us to the idea that medicine is an art and that doctors can be fallible and taught us that we must treat the whole person, not just their pathology.

The book would not exist if it weren't for the encouragement and support over the past two years of my wife Bernadette Jiwa and my colleague Tammy McCausland. Let's just say blood, sweat and tears don't quite cover it. Thanks to my editor Bill Harper and proofreader Leanne Wickham for their care and attention to detail. I have had the privilege to work with two talented designers to bring this project to life. Thank you to Reese Spykerman and Kelly Exeter for bringing your particular gifts to the cover, design and layout of the book.

Finally, I want to acknowledge the people who inspired me to write about the art of doctoring—the medical students, our doctors of the future, who can and will make this a better world. We're in safe hands as long as they remember the primary reason for choosing a career in medicine is to care, not just to cure.

# REFERENCES

## INTRODUCTION

1   Richard Smith: It's hard, perhaps impossibly hard, to be a good doctor', The BMJ, 11 June 2012, https://blogs.bmj.com/bmj/2012/06/11/richard-smith-its-hard-perhaps-impossibly-hard-to-be-a-good-doctor/

2   M. Boland, 'What Do People Expect from Their Doctors?', World Health Forum 16, no. 3 (1995): 221–27; discussion 227-247.

3   Alison Siegel, '8 Questions To Ask Yourself Before You Go On A Second Date With Someone', Elite Daily, accessed 10 September 2018, https://www.elitedaily.com/dating/questions-ask-before-second-date/2000498.

4   Anatole Broyard, Intoxicated by My Illness and Other Writings on Life and Death, First (Fawcett, 1993).

5   J.H. Watanabe, T. McInnes, J.D. Hirsch, 'Cost of Prescription–Drug Related Morbidity and Mortality', Annals of Pharmacotherapy, vol. 52, no. 9 (2018), 829–837. doi: 10.1177/1060028018765159

## WHY DO PEOPLE SEEK HEALTHCARE?

6     M. Wooden, 'Time after time: the myth that Australians work longer hours than anyone else' The Conversation [web article] 30 November 2012, http://theconversation.com/time-after-time-the-myth-that-australians-work-longer-hours-than-anyone-else-4519 (accessed 12 September 2018).

7     J. Baxter, M. Gray, and A. Hayes, 'A snapshot of how Australian Families spend their time' Australian Institute of Family Studies [report], https://aifs.gov.au/publications/snapshot-how-australian-families-spend-their-time (accessed 12 September 2018).

8     The sleep habits of an Australian adult population: A report on the 2015 online sleep survey from the Sleep Health Foundation. Jessica Manousakis, Monash University. Available from https://www.sleephealthfoundation.org.au/pdfs/sleep-week/SHF%20Sleep%20Survey%20Report_2015_final.pdf

9     R.D. Putnam, 'better together: the report of the saguaro seminar: civic engagement in America' 2000 [report], (accessed 23 September 2018). 'Better Together: Report of the Saguaro Seminar on Civic Engagement in America', 2000.

10    Deborah J Schofield et al., 'Premature Retirement Due to Ill Health and Income Poverty: A Cross-Sectional Study of Older Workers', *BMJ Open 3* (2 May 2013), https://doi.org/10.1136/bmjopen-2013-002683.

11    Australian Institute of Health and Welfare, *Australia's Welfare 2009: The Ninth Biennial Welfare Report of the Australian Institute of Health and Welfare.* (Canberra: Australian Institute of Health and Welfare, 2009).

12    Marc Suhrcke, et al., 'Chronic Disease: An Economic Perspective' (Oxford Health Alliance, 2006), http://www.who.int/management/

programme/ncd/Chronic-disease-an-economic-perspective.
pdf.

13   'The Ecology of Medical Care Revisited | NEJM', accessed
     15 September 2018, https://www.nejm.org/doi/pdf/10.1056/
     NEJM200106283442611.

14   Helena Britt, Lisa Valenti, and Graeme Miller, 'Debunking
     the Myth That General Practice Is '6 Minute Medicine'',
     *Byte from the Bettering the Evaluation of Care of Health*
     (BEACH) 2014, no. 002 (2014): 4.

15   Duncan Jake Topliss and Shui Boon Soh, 'Use and Misuse of
     Thyroid Hormone', *Singapore Medical Journal* 54, no. 7 (July
     2013): 406–10; Victor Herbert, 'The Vitamin Craze', *Archives
     of Internal Medicine* 140, no. 2 (1 February 1980): 173–76,
     https://doi.org/10.1001/archinte.1980.00330140031014.

16   Noah J. Switzer, Richdeep S. Gill, and Shahzeer Karmali,
     'The Evolution of the Appendectomy: From Open to
     Laparoscopic to Single Incision', Research article, Scientifica,
     2012, https://doi.org/10.6064/2012/895469.

17   Michael Fitzpatrick, 'Why Can't the Daily Mail Eat
     Humble Pie over MMR?', *BMJ* 331, no. 7525 (10 November
     2005): 1148, https://doi.org/10.1136/bmj.331.7525.1148.

18   Sarah W. Chan et al., 'Montgomery and Informed Consent:
     Where Are We Now?', *BMJ* 357 (12 May 2017): j2224,
     https://doi.org/10.1136/bmj.j2224.

19   'Breast Cancer and Hormone-Replacement Therapy in
     the Million Women Study', *The Lancet* 362, no. 9382 (9
     August 2003): 419–27, https://doi.org/10.1016/S0140-
     6736(03)14065-2.

20   S. F. Brewster, S. Nicholson, and J. R. Farndon, 'The Varicose

Vein Waiting List: Results of a Validation Exercise.', *Annals of The Royal College of Surgeons of England* 73, no. 4 (July 1991): 223–26.

## THE DOCTOR'S WORLD

21    Devesh Oberoi et al., 'Help-seeking Experiences of Men Diagnosed with Colorectal Cancer: A Qualitative Study', *European Journal of Cancer Care* 25, no. 1 (2014), https://onlinelibrary.wiley.com/doi/abs/10.1111/ecc.12271.

22    Moyez Jiwa et al., 'How Do General Practitioners Manage Patients with Cancer Symptoms? A Video-Vignette Study', *BMJ Open* 5, no. 9 (14 September 2015): e008525, https://doi.org/10.1136/bmjopen-2015-008525.

23    M. Jiwa et al., 'Less Haste More Speed: Factors That Prolong the Interval from Presentation to Diagnosis in Some Cancers', *Family Practice* 21, no. 3 (1 June 2004): 299–303, https://doi.org/10.1093/fampra/cmh314.

24    Gemma Ossolinski, Moyez Jiwa, and Alexandra McManus, 'Weight Management Practices and Evidence for Weight Loss through Primary Care: A Brief Review', *Current Medical Research and Opinion* 31, no. 11 (November 2015): 2011–20, https://doi.org/10.1185/03007995.2015.1082993.

25    Nick Goodwin, Natasha Curry, Chris Naylor, Shilpa Ross, and Wendy Duldig, 'Managing people with long-term conditions.' The King's Fund accessed 15 October 2018, https://www.kingsfund.org.uk/sites/default/files/field/field_document/managing-people-long-term-conditions-gp-inquiry-research-paper-mar11.pdf.

26    'How Patient's Unmet Needs Impact Their Health

and Health Care: Highly Cited Difficulties Affording
Prescriptions, Nutritious Food, Transportation Relate
Directly to Health Issues', ScienceDaily, accessed
16 September 2018, https://www.sciencedaily.com/
releases/2015/12/151209183515.htm.

27    Kelly B. Haskard Zolnierek and M. Robin DiMatteo,
      'Physician Communication and Patient Adherence
      to Treatment: A Meta-Analysis', *Medical Care* 47, no.
      8 (August 2009): 826–34, https://doi.org/10.1097/
      MLR.0b013e31819a5acc.

28    M. Song and E. Giovanucci, 'Preventable Incidence and
      Mortality of Carcinoma Associated With Lifestyle Factors
      Among White Adults in the United States.', *JAMA Oncology*
      2, no. 9 (2016): 1154–61.

## THE THEATRE MODEL©

29    Moyez Jiwa et al., 'Rating General Practitioner Consultation
      Performance in Cancer Care: Does the Specialty of
      Assessors Matter? A Simulated Patient Study', *BMC
      Family Practice* 15 (13 September 2014): 152, https://doi.
      org/10.1186/1471-2296-15-152.

30    J.H. Watanabe, T. McInnes, J.D. Hirsch, 'Cost of
      Prescription–Drug Related Morbidity and Mortality', *Annals
      of Pharmacotherapy*, vol. 52, no. 9 (2018), 829–837. doi:
      10.1177/1060028018765159

31    'Imhotep', Ancient History Encyclopedia, accessed 16
      September 2018, https://www.ancient.eu/imhotep/.

32    James McCormick, *The Doctor: Father Figure or Plumber*
      (London: Croom Helm, 1979).

## THE PATIENT (ACTOR 1)

33  '2018 World Population Data Sheet With Focus on Changing Age Structures – Population Reference Bureau', accessed 16 September 2018, https://www.prb.org/2018-world-population-data-sheet-with-focus-on-changing-age-structures/.

34  'Increase in the Median Age of the Population for Selected Countries, 1950-2100 | READ Online', OECD iLibrary, accessed 16 September 2018, https://read.oecd-ilibrary.org/finance-and-investment/oecd-pensions-outlook-2014/increase-in-the-median-age-of-the-population-for-selected-countries-1950-2100_pens_outlook-2014-graph1-en.

35  'WHO | Obesity', WHO, accessed 16 September 2018, http://www.who.int/topics/obesity/en/.

36  World Health Organization, 'Preventing Chronic Diseases : A Vital Investment : WHO Global Report' (Geneva: Geneva : World Health Organization, 2005), http://apps.who.int/iris/handle/10665/43314.

37  'The Ecology of Medical Care Revisited | NEJM'.

38  Helena Britt et al., *A Decade of Australian General Practice Activity* 2006-07 to 2015-16., vol. 41, General Practice Series (Sydney University Press, 2016).

39  'Chart Reveals How Much Clothing Sizes Have Changed over the Past 60 Years - and Shows Size 12 Marilyn Monroe Would Be Anything between a 00 and an 8 Today | Daily Mail Online', accessed 16 September 2018, https://www.dailymail.co.uk/femail/article-3198374/Chart-reveals-clothing-sizes-changed-past-60-years-shows-size-12-Marilyn-Monroe-00-8-today.html.

40  'Teenagers - ADF - *Alcohol & Drug Foundation*', accessed 16 September 2018, https://adf.org.au/alcohol-drug-use/teenagers/; 'Alcohol Advertising That Targets the Young', ADF - Alcohol &

Drug Foundation (blog), accessed 16 September 2018, https://adf.org.au/insights/alcohol-advertising-targets-young/.

41    'Teenagers - ADF - *Alcohol & Drug Foundation*'.

42    'Identifying Signs Of Drug Use | Alcohol & Drug Foundation (ADF)', ADF - *Alcohol & Drug Foundation* (blog), accessed 16 September 2018, https://adf.org.au/alcohol-drug-use/teenagers/identifying-drug-use/.

43    S. Patricia Chou et al., 'The Prevalence of Drinking and Driving in the United States, 2001-2002: Results from the National Epidemiological Survey on Alcohol and Related Conditions', *Drug and Alcohol Dependence* 83, no. 2 (28 June 2006): 137–46, https://doi.org/10.1016/j.drugalcdep.2005.11.001.

44    'Third "Have Sex below Legal Age"', 13 August 2006, http://news.bbc.co.uk/2/hi/4784939.stm.

45    'Men Who Watch Pornography Have Small Brains | Boston.Com', accessed 16 September 2018, https://www.boston.com/culture/health/2014/05/30/men-who-watch-pornography-have-small-brains.

46    'Gym Membership Market Analysis - Statistic Brain', accessed 16 September 2018, https://www.statisticbrain.com/gym-membership-statistics/.

47    'Smartphone Daily Usage Time Worldwide 2017 | Statistic', Statista, accessed 16 September 2018, https://www.statista.com/statistics/781692/worldwide-daily-time-spent-on-smartphone/.

48    F. J. He and G. A. MacGregor, 'A Comprehensive Review on Salt and Health and Current Experience of Worldwide

Salt Reduction Programmes', *Journal of Human Hypertension* 23, no. 6 (June 2009): 363–84, https://doi.org/10.1038/jhh.2008.144.

49 'Annual Alcohol Poll 2018: Attitudes and Behaviours', *FARE* (blog), 21 March 2018, http://fare.org.au/annual-alcohol-poll-2018-attitudes-and-behaviours/.

50 Chris Lovato et al., 'Impact of Tobacco Advertising and Promotion on Increasing Adolescent Smoking Behaviours', *Cochrane Database of Systematic Reviews*, no. 3 (2003), https://doi.org/10.1002/14651858.CD003439; Peter Anderson et al., 'Impact of Alcohol Advertising and Media Exposure on Adolescent Alcohol Use: A Systematic Review of Longitudinal Studies', *Alcohol and Alcoholism* 44, no. 3 (1 May 2009): 229–43, https://doi.org/10.1093/alcalc/agn115.

51 James Nicholls, 'Everyday, Everywhere: Alcohol Marketing and Social Media--Current Trends', *Alcohol and Alcoholism* (Oxford, Oxfordshire) 47, no. 4 (August 2012): 486–93, https://doi.org/10.1093/alcalc/ags043.

52 'Position Statement - Alcohol Pricing and Taxation - National Cancer Control Policy', accessed 16 September 2018, https://wiki.cancer.org.au/policy/Position_statement_-_Alcohol_pricing_and_taxation.

53 Becky Freeman, 'Tobacco Tax Rise Will Help Smokers Butt out for Good', The Conversation, accessed 16 September 2018, http://theconversation.com/tobacco-tax-rise-will-help-smokers-butt-out-for-good-16608.

54 Dementia Australia, 'Dementia Statistics', 7 August 2014, https://www.dementia.org.au/statistics.

55 'Heart Disease in Australia | The Heart Foundation', accessed

16 September 2018, https://www.heartfoundation.org.au/
about-us/what-we-do/heart-disease-in-australia.

56    The Heart Foundation, 'High Blood Pressure Statistics', The
Heart Foundation, accessed 16 September 2018, https://
www.heartfoundation.org.au/about-us/what-we-do/heart-
disease-in-australia/high-blood-pressure-statistics.

57    'Facts and Figures - Cancer Council Australia', accessed 16
September 2018, https://www.cancer.org.au/about-cancer/
what-is-cancer/facts-and-figures.html.

58    'WHO | Obesity'.

59    Hchokr, English: *Bronfenbrenner's Ecological Theory of
Development*, 20 November 2012, 20 November 2012, I
made this diagram to illustrate Bronfenbrenner's Ecological
Theory of Development, https://commons.wikimedia.org/
wiki/File:Bronfenbrenner%27s_Ecological_Theory_of_
Development_(English).jpg.

60    'Social Ecological Model', *Wikipedia*, 27 July 2018, https://
en.wikipedia.org/w/index.php?title=Social_ecological_
model&oldid=852178058.

61    Miranda Herron, 'Junk Food Advertising to Kids -
Shopping', *CHOICE*, 4 September 2014, https://www.
choice.com.au/shopping/packaging-labelling-and-
advertising/advertising/articles/junk-food-advertising-to-
kids.

62    Alessandro R. Demaio et al., 'Rural Australians Are
Missing out on Affordable Fresh Food', *The Conversation*,
accessed 16 September 2018, http://theconversation.com/
rural-australians-are-missing-out-on-affordable-fresh-
food-21358; Rebecca Burns, 'Atlanta's Food Deserts Leave

Its Poorest Citizens Stranded and Struggling', *The Guardian*, 17 March 2014, sec. Cities, http://www.theguardian. com/cities/2014/mar/17/atlanta-food-deserts-stranded- struggling-survive.

63    Nassim Khadem, 'How McDonald's Dodged Half a Billion Dollars in Australian Tax', *The Sydney Morning Herald*, 19 May 2015, https://www.smh.com.au/business/the-economy/ how-mcdonalds-dodged-half-a-billion-dollars-in-australian- tax-20150519-gh5b6q.html.

64    Karl Thompson, 'What Percentage of Your Life Will You Spend at Work?', *ReviseSociology*, 16 August 2016, https:// revisesociology.com/2016/08/16/percentage-life-work/.

65    'The Relationship between Job Satisfaction and Health: A Meta-Analysis | Occupational & Environmental Medicine', accessed 16 September 2018, https://oem.bmj.com/ content/62/2/105.short.

66    Keith A. King, Rebecca Vidourek, and Michelle Schwiebert, 'Disordered Eating and Job Stress among Nurses', *Journal of Nursing Management* 17, no. 7 (1 November 2009): 861–69, https://doi.org/10.1111/j.1365-2834.2009.00969.x.

67    Chandra L. Jackson et al., 'Obesity Trends by Industry of Employment in the United States, 2004 to 2011', *BMC Obesity* 3, no. 1 (2 April 2016): 20, https://doi.org/10.1186/ s40608-016-0100-x.

68    Yihao Liu et al., 'Eating Your Feelings? Testing a Model of Employees' Work-Related Stressors, Sleep Quality, and Unhealthy Eating', *The Journal of Applied Psychology* 102, no. 8 (August 2017): 1237–58, https://doi.org/10.1037/ apl0000209.

69    K.J Duffey, B.M Popkin, 'Energy Density, Portion Size, and
      Eating Occasions: Contributions to Increased Energy Intake
      in the United States, 1977–2006', *PLOS Medicine,* June 28,
      2011, https://doi.org/10.1371/journal.pmed.1001050

70    R.L. Street, P.J. Haidet, 'How Well Do Doctors Know
      their Patients? Factors Affecting Physician Understanding
      of Patients' Health Beliefs', *Journal of General Internal
      Medicine*, vol. 26, no. 1, January 2011, pp. 21–27. https://doi.
      org/10.1007/s11606-010-1453-3

71    K Roberts. *Lovemarks: The Future Beyond Brands* (Expanded
      ed.), New York, PowerHouse Books, 2005.

72    'The Saatchi & Saatchi Lovemarks | What Is Your
      Lovemark', accessed 16 September 2018, http://www.saatchi.
      co.za/network/lovemarks/.

73    Daniel Goleman, 'For Many, Turmoil of Aging Erupts
      in the 50's, Studies Find -', The New York Times, 1989,
      https://www.nytimes.com/1989/02/07/science/for-
      many-turmoil-of-aging-erupts-in-the-50-s-studies-find.
      html?pagewanted=all.

74    Erection Changes After 50: The Facts', Psychology Today,
      accessed 16 September 2018, http://www.psychologytoday.
      com/blog/all-about-sex/201205/erection-changes-after-50-
      the-facts.

75    Daniel Goleman, 'For Many, Turmoil of Aging Erupts
      in the 50's, Studies Find -', The New York Times, 1989,
      https://www.nytimes.com/1989/02/07/science/for-
      many-turmoil-of-aging-erupts-in-the-50-s-studies-find.
      html?pagewanted=all.

76    Karen J. Cruickshanks, Terry L. Wiley, Theodore S. Tweed,

Barbara E.K. Klein, Ronald Klein, Julie A. Mares-Perlman, David M. Nondahl, Prevalence of Hearing Loss in Older Adults in Beaver Dam, Wisconsin: The Epidemiology of Hearing Loss Study, *American Journal of Epidemiology*, Volume 148, Issue 9, 1 November 1998, Pages 879–886, https://doi.org/10.1093/oxfordjournals.aje.a009713

77    C. M. McBride, K. M. Emmons, and I. M. Lipkus, 'Understanding the Potential of Teachable Moments: The Case of Smoking Cessation', *Health Education Research* 18, no. 2 (1 April 2003): 156–70, https://doi.org/10.1093/her/18.2.156.

78    Dariush Mozaffarian et al., 'Heart Disease and Stroke Statistics--2015 *Update: A Report from the American Heart Association*', Circulation 131, no. 4 (27 January 2015): e29-322, https://doi.org/10.1161/CIR.0000000000000152.

79    'Who Are You? 7 Facts about the Average Doctor in Australia | Doctorportal', accessed 16 September 2018, https://www.doctorportal.com.au/who-are-you-7-facts-about-the-average-doctor-in-australia/.

80    Sara N. Bleich et al., 'Impact of Physician BMI on Obesity Care and Beliefs', *Obesity* 20, no. 5 (1 May 2012): 999–1005, https://doi.org/10.1038/oby.2011.402.

81    Jay Schwartz, 'The Average BMI in Men', LIVESTRONG.COM, accessed 16 September 2018, https://www.livestrong.com/article/135472-the-average-bmi-men/.

82    'The Average Body Weight for Women | LIVESTRONG.COM', accessed 16 September 2018, https://www.livestrong.com/article/264142-the-average-body-weight-for-women/.

83    Rolando G. Díaz-Zavala et al., 'Effect of the Holiday

Season on Weight Gain: A Narrative Review',
Research article, Journal of Obesity, 2017, https://doi.
org/10.1155/2017/2085136.

84    Daniel Callahan, 'Preventing Disease, Creating Society',
      *Quality Assurance and Utilization Review 1*, no. 4 (1
      November 1986): 124–27, https://doi.org/10.1177/088571
      3X8600100406.

85    JoAna Stallworth and Jeffrey L. Lennon, 'An Interview with
      Dr. Lester Breslow', *American Journal of Public Health* 93, no.
      11 (November 2003): 1803–5.

86    S. Kayman, W. Bruvold, and J. S. Stern, 'Maintenance
      and Relapse after Weight Loss in Women: Behavioral
      Aspects', *The American Journal of Clinical Nutrition* 52, no.
      5 (November 1990): 800–807, https://doi.org/10.1093/
      ajcn/52.5.800.

87    M. C. Fiore et al., 'Methods Used to Quit Smoking in the
      United States. Do Cessation Programs Help?', *JAMA* 263,
      no. 20 (23 May 1990): 2760–65.

88    M. H. Becker, 'The Tyranny of Health Promotion', *Public
      Health Reviews* 14, no. 1 (1986): 15–23.

89    Margaret Schneider Jamner and Daniel Stockols, eds.,
      *Promoting Human Wellness: New Frontiers for Research,
      Practice and Policy* (Berkeley Los Angeles London:
      University of California Press, 2000), https://publishing.
      cdlib.org/ucpressebooks/view?docId=kt4r29q2tg&chunk.
      id=ch04&toc.depth=1&toc.id=ch04&brand=eschol.

90    Sendhil Mullainathan and Eldar Shafir, *Scarcity: Why Having
      Too Little Means So Much* (Times Books, 2014).

91    Moyez Jiwa et al., 'Factors That Impact on the Application

of Guidelines in General Practice: A Review of Medical
Records and Structured Investigation of Clinical Incidents
in Hypertension.', *Quality in Primary Care* 13, no. 4 (2005):
213–20.

92    Anna Gosline, 'Bored to Death: Chronically Bored People
Exhibit Higher Risk-Taking Behavior', Scientific American,
accessed 16 September 2018, https://www.scientificamerican.
com/article/the-science-of-boredom/.

93    'The Doctor Who Drank Infectious Broth, Gave Himself an
Ulcer, and Solved a Medical Mystery | DiscoverMagazine.
Com', accessed 16 September 2018, http://discovermagazine.
com/2010/mar/07-dr-drank-broth-gave-ulcer-solved-
medical-mystery.

94    'Doggone It: Pet Ownership in Australia - Roy
Morgan Research', accessed 16 September 2018, http://
roymorgan.com.au/findings/6272-pet-ownership-in-
australia-201506032349.

95    'It's Raining Cats and Dogs', accessed 16 September 2018,
https://www.smh.com.au/environment/conservation/its-
raining-cats-and-dogs-20130921-2u6lo.html.

96    'Study Finds "life in the Old Dog" for Pet Owners -
Telegraph', accessed 16 September 2018, https://www.
telegraph.co.uk/news/health/news/10976567/Study-finds-
life-in-the-old-dog-for-pet-owners.html.

97    3 November 2003 Heather CatchpoleABC Monday,
'Pet Ownership and Health: The Bad News', item,
3 November 2003, http://www.abc.net.au/science/
articles/2003/11/03/980815.htm.

98    Bradley Smith, 'The "Pet Effect" Health Related Aspects of

Companion', Emergency Care, 2012.

99    Ben Colagiuri, 'Participant Expectancies in Double-
      Blind Randomized Placebo-Controlled Trials: Potential
      Limitations to Trial Validity', *Clinical Trials* 7, no. 3 (1 June
      2010): 246–55, https://doi.org/10.1177/1740774510367916.

100   Millon, Theodore; Paul H. Blaney; Roger D. Davis (1999).
      *Oxford Textbook of Psychopathology*. Oxford University Press
      US. p. 446. ISBN 978-0-19-510307-6.

101   https://www.gov.uk/taking-sick-leave

102   James Curran, 'The Doctor, His Patient and the Illness',
      *BMJ : British Medical Journal* 335, no. 7626 (3 November
      2007): 941, https://doi.org/10.1136/bmj.39384.467928.94.

## THE DOCTOR (ACTOR 2)

103   'Declining Student Resilience: A Serious Problem for
      Colleges', Psychology Today, accessed 17 September
      2018, https://www.psychologytoday.com/blog/freedom-
      learn/201509/declining-student-resilience-serious-problem-
      colleges.

104   'Physicians (per 1,000 People) | Data', The World Bank,
      accessed 17 September 2018, https://data.worldbank.org/
      indicator/sh.med.phys.zs.

105   Pascal Zurn et al., 'Imbalances in the Health Workforce',
      Briefing Paper (World Health Organization, March 2002).

106   Walter W. Rosser, 'The Decline of Family Medicine as a
      Career Choice', *CMAJ* 166, no. 11 (28 May 2002): 1419–20.

107   Mai Stafford and Michael Marmot, 'Neighbourhood
      Deprivation and Health: Does It Affect Us All Equally?',
      *International Journal of Epidemiology* 32, no. 3 (1 June 2003):

357–66, https://doi.org/10.1093/ije/dyg084.

108   Julian Tudor Hart, 'The Inverse Care Law', *The Lancet*,
      Originally published as Volume 1, Issue 7696, 297, no. 7696
      (27 February 1971): 405–12, https://doi.org/10.1016/S0140-
      6736(71)92410-X.

109   Anette Fischer Pedersen and Peter Vedsted, 'Understanding
      the Inverse Care Law: A Register and Survey-Based Study
      of Patient Deprivation and Burnout in General Practice',
      *International Journal for Equity in Health* 13, no. 1 (12
      December 2014): 121, https://doi.org/10.1186/s12939-014-
      0121-3.

110   Mullainathan and Shafir, S*carcity: Why Having Too Little
      Means So Much*.

111   Barbara Starfield, Leiyu Shi, and James Macinko,
      'Contribution of Primary Care to Health Systems and
      Health', *The Milbank Quarterly* 83, no. 3 (1 September 2005):
      457–502, https://doi.org/10.1111/j.1468-0009.2005.00409.x.

112   Georga Cooke et al., 'Common General Practice
      Presentations and Publication Frequency', *Medication*, 2013.

113   Paul Glasziou and Brian Haynes, 'The Paths from Research
      to Improved Health Outcomes', *BMJ Evidence-Based
      Medicine* 10, no. 1 (1 February 2005): 4–7, https://doi.
      org/10.1136/ebm.10.1.4-a.

114   Mark W. Stolar and Endocrine Fellows Foundation Study
      Group, 'Clinical Management of the NIDDM Patient:
      Impact of the American Diabetes Association Practice
      Guidelines, 1985–1993', *Diabetes Care* 18, no. 5 (1 May
      1995): 701–7, https://doi.org/10.2337/diacare.18.5.701.

115   M. Mashru and A. Lant, 'Interpractice Audit of Diagnosis

and Management of Hypertension in Primary Care:
Educational Intervention and Review of Medical Records.',
*BMJ : British Medical Journal* 314, no. 7085 (29 March 1997):
942–46.

116  Kymberley Thorne, Hayley A. Hutchings, and Glyn Elwyn,
'The Effects of the Two-Week Rule on NHS Colorectal
Cancer Diagnostic Services: A Systematic Literature
Review', *BMC Health Services Research* 6, no. 1 (3 April
2006): 43, https://doi.org/10.1186/1472-6963-6-43.

117  Australian Bureau of Statistics, 'Main Features - Health
Service Usage and Experiences of Care', 24 May 2012,
http://www.abs.gov.au/ausstats/abs@.nsf/Lookup/by%20
Subject/1301.0~2012~Main%20Features~Health%20
service%20usage%20and%20experiences%20of%20care~234.

118  'Medical Practitioners Workforce 2015, How Many Medical
Practitioners Are There? - Australian Institute of Health
and Welfare', accessed 17 September 2018, https://www.
aihw.gov.au/reports/workforce/medical-practitioners-
workforce-2015/contents/how-many-medical-practitioners-
are-there.

119  Linda Hawes Clever and Gary M. Arsham, 'Physicians' Own
Health—Some Advice for the Advisors', *Western Journal of
Medicine* 141, no. 6 (December 1984): 846–54.

120  John Gabbay and Andrée le May, 'Evidence Based
Guidelines or Collectively Constructed "Mindlines?"
Ethnographic Study of Knowledge Management in Primary
Care', *BMJ : British Medical Journal* 329, no. 7473 (30
October 2004): 1013.

123  Gallay, J., Mosha, D., Lutahakana, E. et al. Appropriateness

of malaria diagnosis and treatment for fever episodes according to patient history and anti-malarial blood measurement: a cross-sectional survey from Tanzania. Malar J 17, 209 (2018) doi:10.1186/s12936-018-2357-7

121 Malcolm Forsythe, Michael Calnan, and Barbara Wall, 'Doctors as Patients: Postal Survey Examining Consultants and General Practitioners Adherence to Guidelines', *BMJ* 319, no. 7210 (4 September 1999): 605–8, https://doi.org/10.1136/bmj.319.7210.605.

122 Anders Beich, Dorte Gannik, and Kirsti Malterud, 'Screening and Brief Intervention for Excessive Alcohol Use: Qualitative Interview Study of the Experiences of General Practitioners', *BMJ* 325, no. 7369 (19 October 2002): 870, https://doi.org/10.1136/bmj.325.7369.870.

123 'BJ Fogg's Behavior Model', accessed 27 July 2018, http://www.behaviormodel.org/index.html.

124 'Time Spent with GPs on the Decline', Australian Healthcare & Hospitals Association, 14 November 2013, https://ahha.asn.au/news/time-spent-gps-decline.

125 Christopher Harrison et al., 'Multimorbidity', *Australian Family Physician*, 2013.

126 Alexandra L. Connan, 'The Consultation and Physical Examination', Br J Gen Pract 59, no. 564 (1 July 2009): 544–45, https://doi.org/10.3399/bjgp09X453639.

127 Ray Moynihan, Iona Heath, and David Henry, 'Selling Sickness: The Pharmaceutical Industry and Disease Mongering', *BMJ: British Medical Journal* 324, no. 7342 (13 April 2002): 886–91.

128 'Selling Sickness: Pharma Industry Turning Us All Into

Patients', AHRP (blog), 26 October 2006, http://ahrp.
org/selling-sickness-pharma-industry-turning-us-all-into-
patients/.

129  Geoffrey K. Spurling et al., 'Information from
     Pharmaceutical Companies and the Quality, Quantity, and
     Cost of Physicians' Prescribing: A Systematic Review', *PLOS
     Medicine* 7, no. 10 (19 October 2010): e1000352, https://doi.
     org/10.1371/journal.pmed.1000352.

130  Tara F. Bishop, Alex D. Federman, and Salomeh Keyhani,
     'Physicians' Views on Defensive Medicine: A National
     Survey', Archives of Internal Medicine 170, no. 12
     (28 June 2010): 1081–83, https://doi.org/10.1001/
     archinternmed.2010.155.

131  D. A. Davis et al., 'Changing Physician Performance. A
     Systematic Review of the Effect of Continuing Medical
     Education Strategies', *JAMA* 274, no. 9 (6 September 1995):
     700–705.

132  Brian S. Alper et al., 'How Much Effort Is Needed to Keep
     up with the Literature Relevant for Primary Care?', *Journal
     of the Medical Library Association: JMLA* 92, no. 4 (October
     2004): 429–37.

133  G R Langley et al., 'Effect of Nonmedical Factors on Family
     Physicians' Decisions about Referral for Consultation.',
     *CMAJ: Canadian Medical Association Journal* 147, no. 5 (1
     September 1992): 659–66.

134  Anthony Scott et al., 'The Effect of Financial Incentives
     on the Quality of Health Care Provided by Primary
     Care Physicians', The Cochrane Database of Systematic
     Reviews, no. 9 (7 September 2011): CD008451, https://doi.

org/10.1002/14651858.CD008451.pub2.

135  J. Firth-Cozens and J. Greenhalgh, 'Doctors' Perceptions of the Links between Stress and Lowered Clinical Care', *Social Science & Medicine* (1982) 44, no. 7 (April 1997): 1017–22.

136  J. A. Linder et al., 'Time of Day and the Decision to Prescribe Antibiotics., Time of Day and the Decision to Prescribe Antibiotics', JAMA Internal Medicine, *JAMA Internal Medicine* 174, 174, no. 12, 12 (December 2014): 2029, 2029–31, https://doi.org/10.1001/jamainternmed.2014.5225, 10.1001/jamainternmed.2014.5225.

137  John D. Piette and Eve A. Kerr, 'The Impact of Comorbid Chronic Conditions on Diabetes Care', *Diabetes Care* 29, no. 3 (1 March 2006): 725–31, https://doi.org/10.2337/diacare.29.03.06.dc05-2078.

138  Marjorie Kagawa-Singer and Shaheen Kassim-Lakha, 'A Strategy to Reduce Cross-Cultural Miscommunication and Increase the Likelihood of Improving Health Outcomes', *Academic Medicine: Journal of the Association of American Medical Colleges* 78, no. 6 (June 2003): 577–87.

139  Christopher Pearce et al., 'Computers in the New Consultation: Within the First Minute', *Family Practice* 25, no. 3 (1 June 2008): 202–8, https://doi.org/10.1093/fampra/cmn018.

140  Moyez Jiwa et al., 'Primary Care Visits Out-of-Hours. The Case for Skil Mix?', *Journal of Community Nursing* 15, no. 11 (2001): 4–6.

141  'GP Home Visits Halve in a Decade - Telegraph', accessed 17 September 2018, https://www.telegraph.co.uk/news/

uknews/1559001/GP-home-visits-halve-in-a-decade.html.

142  Yvonne McGowan et al., 'Through Doctors' Eyes: A
     Qualitative Study of Hospital Doctor Perspectives on Their
     Working Conditions', *British Journal of Health Psychology* 18,
     no. 4 (November 2013): 874–91, https://doi.org/10.1111/
     bjhp.12037.

143  Wallace Sampson, 'Antiscience Trends in the Rise of the
     "Alternative Medicine" movement', *Annals of the New York
     Academy of Sciences* 775, no. 1 (1 June 1995): 188–97, https://
     doi.org/10.1111/j.1749-6632.1996.tb23138.x.

144  JoAnn E. Manson and Shari S. Bassuk, 'Vitamin and
     Mineral Supplements: What Clinicians Need to Know',
     *JAMA* 319, no. 9 (6 March 2018): 859–60, https://doi.
     org/10.1001/jama.2017.21012.

145  'Physicians as Leaders: What's Missing? | HealthLeaders
     Media', accessed 17 September 2018, https://www.
     healthleadersmedia.com/strategy/physicians-leaders-whats-
     missing.

146  Moyez Jiwa, 'How Patients Can Improve Health Care', *The
     Journal of Health Design* 3, no. 1 (22 March 2018), https://
     www.journalofhealthdesign.com/JHD/article/view/53.

## THE STAGE

147  Kelly Gooch, 'Patients' No. 1 Complaint? Front-Desk
     Staff', Booker's Hospital Review, April 2016, https://
     www.beckershospitalreview.com/hospital-management-
     administration/patients-no-1-complaint-front-desk-staff.html.

148  Allison B. Arneill and Ann Sloan Devlin, 'Perceived Quality
     of Care: The Influence of the Waiting Room Environment',

*Journal of Environmental Psychology* 22, no. 4 (1 December 2002): 345–60, https://doi.org/10.1006/jevp.2002.0274.

149 'The Multi-Billion Dollar Cost of Looking Good', Suncorp, accessed 17 September 2018, https://www.suncorp.com.au/about-us/news/media/cost-of-looking-good.html.

150 'A Recent Study Shows That People Are Willing To Pay More For Good Service | Business Insider', accessed 17 September 2018, https://www.businessinsider.com.au/just-how-important-is-customer-service-australian-customer-insights-study-finds-it-to-be-critical-2011-8.

151 Britt et al., *A Decade of Australian General Practice Activity* 2006-07 to 2015-16.

152 S. Knox et al., 'Locality Matters: The Influence of Geography on General Practice Activity in Australia 1998–2004', in *General Practice Series* No. 17 (Canberra: Australian Institute of Health and Welfare, 2005).

153 Sarah Long and Moyez Jiwa, 'Satisfying the Patient in Primary Care: A Postal Survey Following a Recent Consultation', *Current Medical Research and Opinion* 20, no. 5 (May 2004): 685–89, https://doi.org/10.1185/030079904125003322.

154 '5 Steps to a Successful Reception Desk Design', Love Your Workspace, 17 October 2017, http://www.loveyourworkspace.co.uk/5-steps-successful-reception-desk-design/.

155 Ibid.

156 Tania Moerenhout et al., 'Patient Health Information Materials in Waiting Rooms of Family Physicians: Do Patients Care?', *Patient Preference and Adherence* 7 (2013):

489–97, http://dx.doi.org/10.2147/PPA.S45777.

157   '5 Steps to a Successful Reception Desk Design'. http://www.
      loveyourworkspace.co.uk/5-steps-successful-reception-desk-
      design/

158   'Some Hotel Chains Ditching the Front Desk - Travel -
      Business Travel | NBC News', accessed 17 September 2018,
      http://www.nbcnews.com/id/39854018/ns/travel-business_
      travel/t/some-hotel-chains-ditching-front-desk/#.WIwhtT-
      wDZc.

159   Gooch, 'Patients' No. 1 Complaint? Front-Desk Staff'.
      https://www.beckershospitalreview.com/hospital-
      management-administration/patients-no-1-complaint-
      front-desk-staff.html

160   Gavin J. Andrews, *Primary Health Care: People, Practice, Place*
      (Routledge, 2016).

161   'HealthMint Medical Centre • A WOW Healthcare
      Experience • Cranbourne North', HealthMint, accessed 17
      September 2018, https://www.healthmint.com.au/.

162   E. Hayes, 'GP Receptionists: Their Work and Training.',
      *Health Visitor* 62, no. 4 (April 1989): 117–18.

## THE SCRIPT

163   P. M. Fischer and S. R. Smith, 'The Nature and Management
      of Telephone Utilization in a Family Practice Setting.', *The
      Journal of Family Practice* 8, no. 2 (February 1979): 321–27.

164   Elizabeth A. Patterson Rn, Christopher Del Mar Fracgp,
      and Jake M. Najman Ba(hons), 'Medical Receptionists
      in General Practice: Who Needs a Nurse?', *International
      Journal of Nursing Practice* 6, no. 5 (1 October 2000): 229–36,

https://doi.org/10.1046/j.1440-172x.2000.00213.x.

165 'A Broader Training for Medical Receptionists | British Journal of General Practice', accessed 17 September 2018, https://bjgp.org/content/30/217/490.short.

166 'NHS Direct "failed Dying Three Year-Old" - Telegraph', accessed 17 September 2018, https://www.telegraph.co.uk/news/nhs/10917119/NHS-Direct-failed-dying-three-year-old.html.

167 Moyez Jiwa, 'The Business of Doctoring', *The Australasian Medical Journal* 5, no. 6 (30 June 2012): 329–33, https://doi.org/10.4066/AMJ.2012.1420.

168 Cooke G, Valenti L, Glasziou P, Britt H. Common general practice presentations and publication frequency. *Aust Fam Physician*. 2013 Jan-Feb;42(1-2):65-8. PMID: 2352946

169 Rachael Rettner, 'Top Reason Patients Sue Doctors: Failure To Diagnose | HuffPost', 19 July 2013, https://www.huffingtonpost.com/2013/07/19/reason-patients-sue-doctors-delay-failure_n_3623509.html?guccounter=1.

170 A. Wilson, 'Consultation Length in General Practice: A Review', *The British Journal of General Practice: The Journal of the Royal College of General Practitioners* 41, no. 344 (March 1991): 119–22.

171 Juliet Mavromatis, 'Why Doctors Interrupt | THCB', The Health Care Blog (blog), 12 June 2012, http://thehealthcareblog.com/blog/2012/06/12/why-doctors-interrupt/.

172 'Confidentiality in the Waiting Room: An Observational Study in General Practice | British Journal of General Practice', accessed 17 September 2018, https://bjgp.org/

content/57/539/490.short.

173   Howard B. Beckman, 'The Effect of Physician Behavior on
      the Collection of Data', Annals of Internal Medicine 101, no.
      5 (1 November 1984): 692, https://doi.org/10.7326/0003-
      4819-101-5-692.

174   David Pendleton et al., eds., *The New Consultation:
      Developing Doctor–Patient Communication* (Oxford: Oxford
      University Press, 2003).

175   Teresa Pawlikowska et al., 'Consultation Models', in
      Learning to Consult (Oxford: Radcliffe, 2007), 179–215.

176   Michael Bungay Stainer, *The Coaching Habit : Say Less, Ask
      More & Change the Way You Lead Forever*, 1 edition (Toronto:
      Box of Crayons Press, 2016).

177   Wendy Levinson et al., 'Not All Patients Want to Participate
      in Decision Making', Journal of General Internal Medicine
      20, no. 6 (June 2005): 531–35, https://doi.org/10.1111/
      j.1525-1497.2005.04101.x.

178   Bungay Stainer, *The Coaching Habit : Say Less, Ask More &
      Change the Way You Lead Forever*.

179   Tovia G. Freedman, '"The Doctor Knows Best" Revisited:
      Physician Perspectives', *Psycho-Oncology* 11, no. 4 (1 July
      2002): 327–35, https://doi.org/10.1002/pon.573.

180   E. Heim, 'Job Stressors and Coping in Health Professions',
      *Psychotherapy and Psychosomatics* 55, no. 2–4 (1991): 90–99,
      https://doi.org/10.1159/000288414.

181   Michael Bungay Stanier, *The Coaching Habit: Say Less, Ask
      More & Change the Way You Lead Forever*, 1 edition (Toronto:
      Box of Crayons Press, 2016).

182   C. A. Barry et al., 'Giving Voice to the Lifeworld. More

Humane, More Effective Medical Care? A Qualitative Study
of Doctor-Patient Communication in General Practice',
Social Science & Medicine (1982) 53, no. 4 (August 2001):
487–505.

183   Roger Ruiz-Moral et al., 'Physician-Patient Communication:
A Study on the Observed Behaviours of Specialty Physicians
and the Ways Their Patients Perceive Them', *Patient
Education and Counseling* 64, no. 1–3 (December 2006):
242–48, https://doi.org/10.1016/j.pec.2006.02.010.

184   Niamh Ramsay, Tracey Johnson, and Tony Badrick, 'Diabetic
Patient Adherence to Pathology Request Completion in
Primary Care', *Australian Health Review: A Publication of the
Australian Hospital Association* 41, no. 3 (July 2017): 277–82,
https://doi.org/10.1071/AH16012.

185   Ryen W. White and Eric Horvitz, 'Cyberchondria: Studies
of the Escalation of Medical Concerns in Web Search',
Microsoft Research, 1 November 2008, https://www.
microsoft.com/en-us/research/publication/cyberchondria-
studies-of-the-escalation-of-medical-concerns-in-web-
search/.

186   'Beneficence', The Free Dictionary, accessed 17 September
2018, http://medical-dictionary.thefreedictionary.com/
beneficence.

187   Robert Cialdini, *Pre-Suasion: A Revolutionary Way to Influence
and Persuade.* (California: Simon & Schuster, 2016).

188   Ibid.

189   Paul K. J. Han et al., 'Conceptual Problems in Laypersons'
Understanding of Individualized Cancer Risk: A Qualitative
Study', *Health Expectations: An International Journal of*

*Public Participation in Health Care and Health Policy* 12, no. 1 (March 2009): 4–17, https://doi.org/10.1111/j.1369-7625.2008.00524.x.

## THE PROPS

190  TEDx Talks, TEDxMaastricht - Fred Lee - 'Patient Satisfaction or Patient Experience ?', accessed 17 September 2018, https://www.youtube.com/watch?v=tylvc9dY400.

191  Moyez Jiwa, 'Deploy Tools That Are Essential to the Office and Alchemy of Healing', *The Journal of Health Design* 1, no. 3 (17 January 2017), https://www.journalofhealthdesign.com/JHD/article/view/18.

192  Moyez Jiwa et al., 'Impact of the Presence of Medical Equipment in Images on Viewers' Perceptions of the Trustworthiness of an Individual On-Screen', *Journal of Medical Internet Research* 14, no. 4 (2012): e100, https://doi.org/10.2196/jmir.1986.

193  Thorin Klosowski, 'How Can I Communicate Better at the Office?', Lifehacker, accessed 17 September 2018, https://lifehacker.com/how-can-i-communicate-better-at-the-office-1001505647.

194  'Why Space Matters: Design as a Driver of Collaboration & Innovation', DesignIntelligence, 9 May 2016, https://www.di.net/articles/why-space-matters-design-as-a-driver-of-collaboration-innovation/.

195  'Body Language - Maximize The Impact Of Seating Formations', accessed 17 September 2018, http://westsidetoastmasters.com/resources/book_of_body_language/chap17.html.

196  Jiwa, Moyez; Krejany, Catherine; Gaedtke, Lee; Kanjo, Epi;
     Nagendran, Ruthra; O'Shea, Carolyn; and Greenlees, Iain
     (2019) "Can doctors improve the patient experience by
     rearranging the furniture and equipment in their office? A
     video recorded simulation," Patient Experience Journal: Vol.
     6 : Iss. 1 , Article 6.
     DOI: 10.35680/2372-0247.1343 Available at: https://
     pxjournal.org/journal/vol6/iss1/6

197  Kelli J Swayden et al., 'Effect of Sitting vs. Standing on
     Perception of Provider Time at Bedside: A Pilot Study',
     *Patient Education and Counseling* 86 (29 June 2011): 166–71,
     https://doi.org/10.1016/j.pec.2011.05.024.

198  Howard Ehrlichman and Jack Halpern, 'Affect and Memory:
     Effects of Pleasant and Unpleasant Odors on Retrieval of
     Happy and Unhappy Memories.', *Journal of Personality and
     Social Psychology* 55, no. 5 (1988): 769–79.

199  https://fortune.com/2019/11/30/science-behind-scent-
     marketing-brand-smells/.

200  Gordon M. Shepherd, 'The Human Sense of Smell: Are We
     Better than We Think?', *PLoS Biology* 2, no. 5 (2004): 146,
     https://doi.org/10.1371/journal.pbio.0020146.

201  'https://fortune.com/2019/11/30/science-behind-scent-
     marketing-brand-smells/.'.

202  Suzy Strutner, 'Airlines Infuse Planes With Smells To Calm
     You Down (And Make You Love Them)', 26 March 2015,
     https://www.huffingtonpost.com.au/entry/airlines-infuse-
     planes-with-smells-to-calm-you-down-and-make-you-love-
     them_us_551028d0e4b01b796c526510.

203  'The Power of Touch | The New Yorker', accessed 17

September 2018, https://www.newyorker.com/science/maria-konnikova/power-touch.

204 Carter Singh and Drew Leder, 'Touch in the Consultation', *British Journal of General Practice* 62, no. 596 (2012): 147–48, https://doi.org/10.3399/bjgp12X630133.

205 Brian Murray, Gore Marina, and Leonard Nicole, 'Impact of Traditional Versus Flavored Tongue Depressors on Pediatric Oropharynx Exam', *Clinical Pediatrics* 57, no. 9 (2018): 1053–57, https://doi.org/10.1177/0009922817743572.

206 Miguel Alonso-Alonso et al., 'Food Reward System: Current Perspectives and Future Research Needs', *Nutrition Reviews* 73, no. 5 (2015): 296–307, https://doi.org/10.1093/nutrit/nuv002.

207 Brown, K. W., & Moskowitz, D. S. (1997). Does unhappiness make you sick? The role of affect and neuroticism in the experience of common physical symptoms. *Journal of Personality and Social Psychology*, 72(4), 907-917. http://dx.doi.org/10.1037/0022-3514.72.4.907

## THE ACTION

208 L. A. Green et al., 'The Ecology of Medical Care Revisited', *The New England Journal of Medicine* 344, no. 26 (28 June 2001): 2021–25, https://doi.org/10.1056/NEJM200106283442611.

209 P. Hjortdahl and C. F. Borchgrevink, 'Continuity of Care: Influence of General Practitioners' Knowledge about Their Patients on Use of Resources in Consultations.', *BMJ* 303, no. 6811 (9 November 1991): 1181–84, https://doi.org/10.1136/bmj.303.6811.1181.

210   Matthew J Ridd, Diana L Santos Ferreira, Alan A
      Montgomery, Chris Salisbury, and William Hamilton,
      'Patient–doctor continuity and diagnosis of cancer: electronic
      medical records study in general practice,' *Br J Gen Pract* 65,
      no. 634 (May 2015): e305-e311, https://doi.org/10.3399/
      bjgp15X684829.

211   Susan L. Ettner, 'The Relationship Between Continuity of
      Care and the Health Behaviors of Patients: Does Having a
      Usual Physician Make a Difference?', *Medical Care* 37, no. 6
      (June 1999): 547.

212   Richelle J. Koopman et al., 'Continuity of Care
      and Recognition of Diabetes, Hypertension, and
      Hypercholesterolemia', *Archives of Internal Medicine* 163,
      no. 11 (9 June 2003): 1357–61, https://doi.org/10.1001/
      archinte.163.11.1357.

213   D A Christakis et al., 'The Association between Greater
      Continuity of Care and Timely Measles-Mumps-Rubella
      Vaccination.', *American Journal of Public Health* 90, no. 6
      (June 2000): 962–65.

214   Koopman, Richelle J., Arch G. Mainous III, Richard
      Baker, James M. Gill, and Gregory E. Gilbert,. 'Continuity
      of care and recognition of diabetes, hypertension, and
      hypercholesterolemia,' *Archives of internal medicine* 163, no.
      11 (2003): 1357-1361.

215   Valerie Beral, Emily Banks, and Gillian Reeves, 'Evidence
      from Randomised Trials on the Long-Term Effects of
      Hormone Replacement Therapy', *The Lancet* 360, no. 9337
      (21 September 2002): 942–44, https://doi.org/10.1016/
      S0140-6736(02)11032-4.

216  John Canton, Kate M Scott, and Paul Glue, 'Optimal
     Treatment of Social Phobia: Systematic Review and Meta-
     Analysis', *Neuropsychiatric Disease and Treatment* 8 (2012):
     203–15, https://doi.org/10.2147/NDT.S23317.

217  Susan A. Abookire et al., 'Use and Monitoring of Statin
     Lipid-Lowering Drugs Compared With Guidelines',
     *Archives of Internal Medicine* 161, no. 1 (8 January 2001):
     53–58, https://doi.org/10.1001/archinte.161.1.53.

218  A. P. Sempere et al., 'Neuroimaging in the Evaluation of
     Patients with Non-Acute Headache', *Cephalalgia* 25, no. 1
     (1 January 2005): 30–35, https://doi.org/10.1111/j.1468-
     2982.2004.00798.x.

219  D. Kendrick et al., 'The Role of Radiography in Primary
     Care Patients with Low Back Pain of at Least 6 Weeks
     Duration: A Randomised (Unblinded) Controlled Trial',
     *Health Technology Assessment* (Winchester, England) 5, no. 30
     (2001): 1–69.

220  Genevieve Cadieux et al., 'Predictors of Inappropriate
     Antibiotic Prescribing among Primary Care Physicians',
     *CMAJ* 177, no. 8 (9 October 2007): 877–83, https://doi.
     org/10.1503/cmaj.070151.

221  Gregory W. Froehlich and H. Gilbert Welch, 'Meeting
     Walk-in Patients' Expectations for Testing Effects on
     Satisfaction', *Journal of General Internal Medicine* 11, no.
     8 (1 August 1996): 470–74, https://doi.org/10.1007/
     BF02599041.

222  Jiwa et al., 'How Do General Practitioners Manage Patients
     with Cancer Symptoms?'

223  Moyez Jiwa et al., 'Implementing Referral Guidelines:

Lessons from a Negative Outcome Cluster Randomised
Factorial Trial in General Practice', *BMC Family Practice* 7,
no. 1 (2 November 2006): 65, https://doi.org/10.1186/1471-
2296-7-65.

224 Moyez Jiwa et al., 'Impact of Referral Letters on Scheduling
of Hospital Appointments: A Randomised Control Trial',
*The British Journal of General Practice* 64, no. 624 (July 2014):
e419–25, https://doi.org/10.3399/bjgp14X680509.

225 Paul Glasziou and Brian Haynes, 'Editorial: The Paths from
Research to Improved Health Outcomes', *ACP Journal Club*
142, no. 2 (2005): A8, https://doi.org/doi:10.7326/ACPJC-
2005-142-2-A08.

226 Paul J. Zak, Robert Kurzban, and William T. Matzner, 'The
Neurobiology of Trust', *Annals of the New York Academy
of Sciences* 1032 (December 2004): 224–27, https://doi.
org/10.1196/annals.1314.025.

227 Steven D. Pearson and Lisa H. Raeke, 'Patients' Trust in
Physicians: Many Theories, Few Measures, and Little Data',
*Journal of General Internal Medicine* 15, no. 7 (1 July 2000):
509–13, https://doi.org/10.1046/j.1525-1497.2000.11002.x.

228 'Why Do Some Companies Thrive While Others Fail?
| Stanford Graduate School of Business', accessed 17
September 2018, https://www.gsb.stanford.edu/insights/
why-do-some-companies-thrive-while-others-fail.

229 'Australian Commission on Safety and Quality in Health
Care Launches First Australian Atlas of Healthcare
Variation | Safety and Quality', accessed 17 September
2018, https://www.safetyandquality.gov.au/media_releases/
australian-commission-on-safety-and-quality-in-health-

care-launches-first-australian-atlas-of-healthcare-variation/.

230   Starfield, Shi, and Macinko, 'Contribution of Primary Care
      to Health Systems and Health'.

231   Felicity Goodyear-Smith and Bob Mash, International
      Perspectives on Primary Care Research (CRC Press, 2017).

**CONCLUSION**

232   Issie Lapowsky, 'Paul Graham on Building Companies for
      Fast Growth', https://www.inc.com/magazine/201309/issie-
      lapowsky/how-paul-graham-became-successful.html .

233   H. M. Swick, 'Toward a Normative Definition of Medical
      Professionalism', *Academic Medicine: Journal of the Association
      of American Medical Colleges* 75, no. 6 (June 2000): 612–16.

234   'Projection of Australian Health Care Expenditure by
      Disease, 2003 to 2033, Table of Contents', Australian
      Institute of Health and Welfare, accessed 17 September
      2018, https://www.aihw.gov.au/reports/health-welfare-
      expenditure/projection-of-australian-health-care-
      expenditure-b/contents/table-of-contents.

235   'Alexander Osterwalder', Better Practice, accessed 17
      September 2018, http://betterpractice.org/index.php/author/
      alexander-osterwalder/.

www.ingramcontent.com/pod-product-compliance
Lightning Source LLC
Chambersburg PA
CBHW020252030426
42336CB00010B/720